BETTER
SEX
THROUGH
YOGA

BETTER
SEX
THROUGH
YOGA

Easy Routines to **Boost Your**

Sex Drive, Enhance Physical **Pleasure,**

and **Spice Up Your Bedroom Life**

Jacquie Noelle Greaux, Jennifer Langheld, and Garvey Rich
Photographs by **Garvey Rich**

Broadway Books

New York

PUBLISHED BY BROADWAY BOOKS

Copyright © 2007 by Yoga Craze LLC

All Rights Reserved

Published in the United States by Broadway Books, an imprint of The Doubleday Broadway Publishing Group, a division of Random House, Inc., New York. www.broadwaybooks.com

BROADWAY BOOKS and its logo, a letter B bisected on the diagonal, are trademarks of Random House, Inc.

For photo credits, see page 269.

This book is not intended to take the place of medical advice from a trained medical professional. Readers are advised to consult a physician or other qualified health professional regarding treatment of their medical problems. Neither the publisher nor the author takes any responsibility for any possible consequences from any treatment, action, or application of medicine, herb, or preparation to any person reading or following the information in this book.

Photographs by Garvey Rich

Library of Congress Cataloging-in-Publication Data
Greaux, Jacquie Noelle.
   Better sex through yoga : easy routines to boost your sex drive, enhance physical pleasure, and spice up your bedroom life / Jacquie Noelle Greaux, Jennifer Langheld, and Garvey Rich ; Photographs by Garvey Rich. — 1st ed.
      p.   cm.
   1. Sex instruction.   2. Sex.   3. Yoga.   I. Langheld, Jennifer.   II. Rich, Garvey.
III. Title.
   HQ31.G77   2007
   613.9'6—dc22

                                                                          2006033300

ISBN 978-0-7679-2058-2

PRINTED IN THE UNITED STATES OF AMERICA

10   9   8   7   6   5   4   3   2   1

First Edition

To all those who know the truth and are willing to share it

CONTENTS

Standing Poses

Duo Assisted Poses

Sexy Secretary Poses

5 CORE ROUTINES 214

BETTER

SEX

THROUGH

YOGA

THIS AIN'T NO TANTRA, BABY

If you've ever done it, or seen people doing it, then you know. Yoga is sexy. While you're bent over backward with your hips thrusting forward, or if you've seen someone at the gym upside-down, with her firm backside tilted in your direction, then you've probably felt a little tingling . . . down there. Yoga even *looks* sexy: with the skimpy clothes, graceful moves, heavy breathing, and sweat. Maybe you've pranced around after class, feeling like a seductive millionaire. Or maybe you remember when our favorite vixen from *Sex in the City,* Samantha Jones, coined the catchy phrase "yogasm" to describe her encounters with male classmates after her yoga class. Wouldn't it be fun to bring all of that yoga sexiness into your bedroom? We think we've discovered how.

It's *Better Sex Through Yoga,* our unique program designed not only to jump-start your libido but also to get you sexually fit. It's for singles looking to hone their bedroom skills and couples wanting to reignite the flame. It's for any woman who fears she's lost touch with herself "down there" and wants to reconnect with her sexuality in a fun, sexy way. And whether you're young or old, big or small, a seasoned yogi looking for an exciting twist to your practice or a yoga virgin interested in a new, simple way to become more sexually—and physically—fit, this book is for you. You'll wind up with an awesome new body, but the best benefits will be something only you and your partner will be able to experience: amazing new lovemaking skills. Just think of us as your *very* personal trainer.

Most books about yoga and sex focus on Tantric sex. Tantra is, by definition, about discovering and stimulating sensual spirituality and being one with one's surroundings. Tantra teaches practitioners how to discover energy for sexual pleasure, for bringing joy and wholeness to everyday life, and for aiding in spiritual evolution. Tantra yoga includes visualization, chanting, and strong breathing practices. Books presenting principles of Tantric sex offer sex positions from the Kama Sutra meant to create a stronger connection with your partner. We're not exactly Tantra. However, our *Better Sex Through Yoga* program can be the perfect complement to what you'll find there—or it can stand on its own.

We're always looking for ways to improve our sex lives. Countless magazines and ads pitch us products and gizmos that promise better sex. But we've discovered that the secret lies right on our yoga mats! Even the simplest *Better Sex Through Yoga* moves can empower your sexual and creative vitality in a mind-blowing way. We'll just tease you with a few examples of what we're talking about. Practicing our Cha-Cha-Cha move will translate into the hot Latin-loving hip moves in bed. The Sexy Secretary routine is perfect for tight hips and bad posture from sitting all day. Between the Sheets is a "quickie" routine before the quickie with your lover—done in bed, delivering flexibility and fun for those of us with inflexible schedules. Whether at the office, before a hot date, or during a five-minute quickie, this book's goal is to keep you sexually fit—in both mind and body.

By investing just a little time every week, you can become a powerful erotic force capable of reducing your lucky partner to a state of gasping, spent gratitude. We've pulled together traditional yoga poses as well as some yoga-inspired moves specifically created to skyrocket your sexual appetite. Even learning to assist your partner while he practices yoga can be quite the natural aphrodisiac. Best of all, you'll find that you're able to achieve heights of pleasure that you've never reached before. All you have to do is tap in to your body's vast network of pleasure points—also known as your sexual core (lots more about this later).

Without proper maintenance, your sexual core can crash. *Better Sex Through Yoga* offers routines that, when practiced regularly, will repair, restore, and rejuvenate your sexual core. Trust us, results are immediate.

Not only will you learn and discover new exciting sex positions, but also you'll find yourself feeling friskier throughout the day. Your increased strength, along with enhanced flexibility and, best of all, a sexual core awakening, will send you on your way to an amazing sex life. And don't worry; you don't need to be a contortionist to get instant sexual benefits. There are no complicated positions to master—just simple yet highly effective moves that will shape you up where it matters most: in the bedroom.

1

FIRST A LITTLE FOREPLAY

Sex, as we all know, is more than just the act of having sex. It's about a whole experience that begins with an exciting warm-up called foreplay. With foreplay, you begin to build excitement as blood starts to rush throughout your body and tingle every nook and cranny of your sexual being. As you start to kiss and touch and gently explore your partner's sensual areas, your pleasure zones start to kick into high gear. Ultimately, foreplay helps to set the mood for the lovemaking that's soon to come.

Why Yoga?

Like foreplay, we'd like to set the mood for *Better Sex Through Yoga* by explaining how our program got off the ground. As you probably realize, the basis for *Better Sex Through Yoga* is of course *yoga*. We start with yoga because so many of its principles simply and readily apply to sex. Over our years of teaching and practicing yoga, we've found that it is incredibly suited for waking up your body, mind, and spirit to help you achieve a better sex life.

Yoga has been around for thousands of years (clearly not as long as people have been having sex but well before we started teaching *Better Sex Through Yoga*). Over time, yoga has evolved into an amazing practice that promotes not only physical development but mental, emotional, and spiritual development as well. Although there are many different styles and forms of yoga, all these different forms have in common some basic yoga principles. We've chosen ten of these powerful yoga principles to incorporate into our *Better Sex Through Yoga* program. Here's how:

1. COMPASSION

The yoga principle of compassion is often referred to as nonviolence. But we take it to mean something more than just not hurting—or killing—another person. Compassion, for us, is about your ability to love and be loved. Loving not just yourself but everyone around you. Most important, from this yoga principle, you want to cultivate your compassion—and love—at many different levels. The compassion developed by practicing yoga leads to better sex. Can you have great sex without love and compassion? Yes, you might end up with a quickie or night or two of passionate lovemaking, but for sustained better sex, first you'll need to cultivate compassion and love for others.

2. BODY OF KNOWLEDGE

Through yoga, you'll gain intimate knowledge of your own body while getting an amazing workout. You'll learn to understand what feels good and what doesn't and how to tweak a pose for better results or when to cool it and rest. This understanding of your own body and your energy of that day will make you a better yogi—yoga practitioner—and a better lover. One teacher had a favorite expression: "A new body everyday." Get to know your body and check in each day. Discovering that you may have more sexual desire and looser hips will make for a very romantic evening.

3. MOVEMENT

Yoga is about moving your body gracefully and really understanding how moving can affect all aspects of your life. Many of the seemingly small, subtle movements that you practice in yoga, such as tilting your pelvis and breathing into certain body parts, can be very useful—and pleasurable—for lovemaking.

4. GRACE UNDER PRESSURE

The breath and linking your breath to movement is one of the main principles of yoga. As you practice the different *Better Sex Through Yoga* poses, you'll learn how to breathe freely and deeply while your body is under physical stress. Most of the time, sex is a great release of tension—sexual, physical, and emotional—but sometimes sex itself can be stressful. Are you trying too hard to achieve orgasm? When stresses and pressures arise in the bedroom, let your breath release those tensions to help you focus on the pleasure of sex itself.

5. FLEX IT UP

If you've ever stopped working out, the first thing you probably noticed is that your body stiffened and tightened up. The natural process of aging also does this to your body. You might have even felt pain in opening your legs or bending backward when your lover is going down on you. The physical movements of yoga help to free your body and become more flexible where it really counts: in the bedroom.

6. STRENGTH

Practicing yoga brings strength to your entire body. When you're weak and tired, your body feels heavy and sluggish. It's like dragging around a heavy weight that you can't get rid of. As you build strength through yoga, your body will start to feel as if it's lifting off the ground. That sensation of lightness will transform all of your everyday experiences—most important, sex. Not only will you be able to last longer, but you might be able to literally sweep your partner off his feet. Being physically strong will allow you to move yourself and your lover around with ease and will take your lovemaking to a whole new level.

7. AWARENESS

Awareness is about being present in what you're doing now; it means focusing on the moment and not letting your mind wander off, which can happen during both sex and exercise. With *Better Sex Through Yoga*, we stress that you stay present and focus on the yoga pose at hand. The same holds true for the bedroom; stay in the moment.

8. INNER TRUE HAPPINESS

Okay, we're not saying that great sex can't make you happy. But just as yoga teaches that true happiness comes from within, eventually you'll want to move beyond the immediate gratification of a terrific orgasm. Once you've mastered the techniques of *Better Sex Through Yoga*, you'll find that great sex is just the beginning of a more fulfilling life.

9. FAKE IT TILL YOU MAKE IT

If you've ever felt overwhelmed, awkward, or simply unmotivated by the thought of exercising or making love, just do it. More often than not, once you begin, your body's natural desire and motivation will kick into high gear. Likewise, if a position—either on the mat or between the sheets—seems too daunting, just give a try. You'll end up loving it. Remember, instant perfection isn't the goal here; feeling good and increasing your sexual satisfaction is.

10. BURNING ENTHUSIASM

This yoga principle is all about the disciplined use of energy, which literally translates as fire and heat. We want you to bring a renewed sense of passion and conviction to having sex, not just to go through the motions and lie there like a log as your partner gets off. Ignite your fire and bring passion to your sex life! *Better Sex Through Yoga* poses will add that spark—your job is just to keep the flame alive.

Why Sex Through Yoga Is Better

Now you know how the basic yoga principles are a good starting point for you to improve your sex life. But we wanted to take yoga poses a step further to really help you focus on having better sex. To that end, we've combined the poses in this book with some other types of exercise and movement programs. We've carefully considered the benefits that many different types of mind/body techniques, practices, and postures have on your body—and your sex life—and have come up with this new equation for better sex:

Yoga + Pilates + Chakra Balancing + Dance
= Your Ticket to a New Sex Life!

Yoga

Yoga is the foundation of the *Better Sex Through Yoga* practice, offering strength, stamina, flow, proper breathing, and sexual core control.

Pilates

With an emphasis on your core abdominal muscles (abs), *Better Sex Through Yoga* expands on Pilates techniques with a deeper waking up, strengthening, and relaxing of your sexual core. Pilates is a system of original exercises developed by Joseph Pilates for strengthening your core in a safe way. Some of the exercises are done on the floor (mat work) while others are done on special Pilates exercise equipment. An intelligent style of movement, Pilates is now used preventively by dancers, athletes, and others to help stave off injuries. Dancers are perhaps more aware than most people that a strong core is critical for grace, strength, and stamina—all important for great sex too.

Chakra Balancing

Like acupressure points, chakras are energy centers located throughout your body that transmit and receive energy called *chi* (more about this in Chapter 3). When you are sick or perhaps just don't feel like having sex, your chakras might be out of balance—meaning that energy—including sexual energy—can't flow properly. Yoga helps to realign the chakras and stimulate energy flow throughout your entire body for optimum pleasure.

Dance

Better Sex Through Yoga routines are influenced by the style and fluidity that dance pioneers are known for. We've mixed a bit of ballet and hip-hop into our routines to keep them playful, sexy, and graceful. Extension and precision of movement, done while looking perfectly at ease, are essential for the dancer . . . and the yogi alike.

=

Better Sex Through Yoga is unique in that we embrace the sexual benefits of yoga. Most yoga practices offer mind and body balance; *Better Sex Through Yoga*, however, focuses on mind and body *pleasure*. We combine the concept of better sex and yoga through simple and nontraditional instruction with actual how-to sex positions that you can practice while in bed, in the tub, or in the car.

And we use actual yoga positions! *Better Sex Through Yoga* offers you actual sex positions that mimic yoga positions found in our routine. Our Bump Bump Bump move (page 86), for example, sends gentle shock waves through your pelvis while giving you killer inner thighs. How does that sound? Once you've mastered this move on the mat, we encourage you to try it in the bedroom.

So why try *Better Sex Through Yoga*? Yes, you want a better sex life, but we can give you twelve other reasons to keep coming back. Here are some of the other great benefits you can expect after practicing *Better Sex Through Yoga*:

1. A "yoga hottie body" with a sexy yoga butt, firm abs, yummy tummy, toned thighs, posture like a dancer, and a traffic-stopping, totally erotic glow
2. More energy, less stress, and an overall "natural high"
3. The ability to discover the power of your sexual core
4. Enhanced range of motion in your hips and waist
5. Improved coordination and balance for any yoga or sex position
6. Better circulation, especially in the genital area
7. Deeper, longer, better breathing patterns that offer fresh oxygen to the sexual region and heighten sensitivity
8. A rush of endorphins (the feel-good chemicals released throughout the body) after any yoga—or lovemaking—session
9. Greater flexibility and stamina, which leads to more staying power in the bedroom

10. Greater control of your sexual organs in relation to the rest of your body
11. Deeper, more powerful and intense orgasms
12. A sexier, more confident you in the bedroom—and beyond

Enough foreplay. You see why we're so excited for you to get started. Next we'll test your sexual fitness and see how you measure up.

2

WHAT IS YOUR SEXUAL FITNESS?

Now that you understand why we've created *Better Sex Through Yoga,* it's time to consider your fitness level. Don't worry, it's not about how many push-ups you can do or how fast you can run a mile; we're talking about your sexual fitness.

Sexual fitness is simple: It's a measure of your sexual satisfaction and sexual pleasure. Just like any kind of fitness, it has levels from beginner to advanced (the level you'll reach after practicing our fabulous *Better Sex Through Yoga* routines). It doesn't matter if you have sex seven times a week or seven times a year—sexual fitness isn't about how much sex you are having, it's about how good it is each time you have it.

Understanding your body sexually is about knowing what feels good and what doesn't, learning which muscles do what and how, and knowing when to contract or relax those muscles. And just like any exercise, this understanding requires conditioning. If your muscles are underused or if you're out of shape, you'll have poor sexual performance. But a sexually fit body will give you amazing stamina during lovemaking and bring you and your partner to new heights of pleasure.

Good Sex Is a Good Thing

Believe it or not, one of the best ways to start improving your sexual fitness is to start having more sex. Just do it! Have more sex and don't be embarrassed or ashamed about it either. It's perfectly natural for you to want sex. Of course, we want you to be safe and thoughtful about whom you have sex with, but the bottom line is that sex is a really good thing, good for your body and for your well-being. And great sex is even better. Here are some healthful reasons to make you want more sex.

Sex Protects You. "Have great sex and call me in the morning." Can you imagine your doctor offering you this prescription as a cure for the common cold? Believe it! Experts have found that sex boosts chemicals in your body that really can protect you against disease. Researchers have found that people who have frequent sex have higher levels of an antibody called Immunoglobulin A, which boosts the immune system and protects against infections. Want to know how to protect against colds and flu this season? Have more sex! What a great concept!

Follow Your Heart. Depending on your level of enthusiasm (and possibly skill), intercourse can be an aerobic exercise, burning up to 200 calories per session. To burn that many calories at the gym, you'd have to jog on the treadmill for twenty to thirty minutes (depending on your level of intensity). According to *Forbes* magazine, British researchers found that by having sex three times a week for a year, you can burn off the equivalent of six Big Macs! But the benefits are bigger than just calorie-burning. Research has also found that men who have sex two times per week have fewer heart attacks than those who do not. Which is great news, and not only for men. Did you know that heart disease is the leading killer of American *women?* One of the best ways to prevent cardiovascular disease is regular exercise, which brings us back to what we were saying about what wonderful, heart-healthy, calorie-burning exercise sex can be.

"Not Tonight, Dear, I've Got a Headache." If you've ever uttered those famous words then you are in for a surprise. Far from being an excuse to abstain, a headache is actually a good reason to *get it on*. (Check out page 249 for our routine.) Orgasm causes your brain to release hormones that can alleviate headaches (even migraines) and also reduce PMS pain, arthritis pain, and lots of other ailments. You've got a headache? Then get busy!

Sexual Healing. *Yes, sex has curative powers!* Remember how those hormones released in your brain during sex can cure headaches and other aches and pains? Those same chemicals can provide another powerful benefit: They can actually help the healing process. It seems incredible, but science is showing that sexual activity can speed the healing of cuts, blisters, and bruises. Swedish scientists found that animals with wounds healed twice as fast when they were injected with sex hormones. And researchers in Ohio have been studying married couples to see how sex helps the healing process in humans. Who knew sex could actually heal? Sure sounds like more fun than a Band-Aid!

Oh, That Afterglow—Sex Gives Hormone Highs. Ladies, listen up! Want to improve your complexion, protect against a whole host of ailments, and even be more attractive to men in the process? Then have more sex! Studies show that women who have more sex have higher levels of estrogen. Estrogen is essential to healthy, smooth, and silky skin. So save a bundle in skin-care products, and go for it!

The benefits go beyond a rosy-cheeked glow. Increases in estrogen also help to protect women from heart disease, osteoporosis, and Alzheimer's disease. Not only that, the more sex you have, the more sex you'll be offered. You are probably wondering how we can know such a thing. It all comes down to science. When we are more sexually active, we give off more pheromones (the chemicals our bodies produce to increase the interest of the opposite sex). So the more you do it, the more opportunities you'll have to do it over (and over and over) again.

Sex Energizes—and Relaxes. When we're stressed out and nervous, we're often advised to take a deep breath in order to relax. Good advice, but maybe we should also be advised to have an orgasm. It's true: Science shows that sex is calming. After orgasm there is a point of extreme mental and physical relaxation—what a great way to prepare for bed!

Yes, sex can help you relax to sleep. But the calming benefits of sex extend beyond sleep. Research shows that the relaxation we experience after orgasm can loosen us not only throughout a night's sleep, but also into our daily lives, helping us cope with stress at work, during public speaking, and so forth.

A study at the University of Paisley in Scotland compared sexually active men and women with their abstinent counterparts. What they found was astonishing. Not only were the sexually active individuals less stressed and more relaxed right after orgasm, but the calming benefits of sex lasted for days at the time!

The More Sex, the Merrier. With increased sexual activity comes increased circulation to all areas of the body, especially the genitalia. This increased circulation stimulates and revitalizes the genitalia nerve endings. Some thrill-seekers eat chili peppers and ginger to stimulate nerve endings and aid orgasm. But the best way to improve the circulation to your genitals and get those nerve endings tingling is simply to have more sex! The more you do it, the better it feels. Isn't life grand?

Work Those Love Muscles

Now you see why sex is so good for you. But as we promised, we want you to have better sex. To do that, you'll need to know some basics about your body to improve your sexual fitness. If they are exercised properly through the *Better Sex Through Yoga* routines, we believe that these *love muscles* can really ignite your sexual prowess and increase your enjoyment of sex.

The love muscles are primarily your hips, butt, thighs, and abdominals, as well as your deep internal sex muscles and organs (your sexual core). Your breath and blood circulation also play a role in keeping those love muscles active and healthy.

Hips. Your hips are of vital importance to your sexual well-being. Stiff hips can cause discomfort during sex by limiting your flexibility and preventing you from holding a particularly pleasurable position. Really tight hips can even diminish your sex drive. Why? Stiff hips constrict blood flow to the sexual region, which diminishes nerve activity and pleasure.

Butt, Thighs, and Abdominals. These muscles aren't there simply to be attractive in your low-rise jeans (until you get a *Better Sex Through Yoga* yoga butt!). They are some of the strongest muscles in your body, providing your power and balance. Tightness or weakness in any of these muscle groups will cause early fatigue during the act of sex, taking you out of the moment. Not being toned in this area can also sap your self-confidence and sexual command. The butt, thighs, and abs are also responsible for your posture and gait, which have a great affect on your sexual confidence. Put simply, when this region is strong, engaged, and working in harmony, you feel great—and look great, even in those leather pants!

Sexual Core. Knowing your body also means plunging deeper into your sexual anatomy, the part that we call your sexual core. The sexual core starts beneath the navel and reaches to the pelvic floor, including the pelvis, hips, abdominals, and a small group of muscles located deep inside the pelvis called the pubococcygeal (don't blame us, we didn't make up the name), or, PC muscles. These muscles in the pelvis play a big role in genital stimulation, sensation, and pleasure. Prolonged sitting, shortened breath, and neglecting to exercise them will weaken these muscles over time. Our subtle *Better Sex Through Yoga* moves instruct you how to squeeze and release internally to deliver pleasure to your partner. Regular practice of these exercises will increase your levels of orgasms and heighten clitoral and penile sensations. You've heard the expression "getting there is half of the fun"?

Guys have PC muscles too and you'll want to tell him about his for his extended pleasure as well as yours. Strong male PC muscles can help achieve and maintain erection as well as delay and prolong orgasm.

The tricky part is, most of us never contract our PC muscles. For one thing, they usually work hard only when we really need to urinate. Other than that, with our sitting for long periods and bad posture and breathing, we often neglect these muscles. We cannot see them contract, but we can certainly feel them.

The easiest way to locate them for the first time is to sit on the toilet, and, while urinating, stop the flow. (Yes, we know this doesn't sound very sexy, but bear with us.) You are seeking to duplicate that same sensation while you are not urinating. Practice squeezing these muscles tightly for about two slow counts, then slowly releasing them for the same time. Contract internally and exhale simultaneously, your lower belly pulling inward, your pelvic floor (the space between your tailbone and pubic bone) contracting. Inhale and release. Do it again. Voilà! These very simple moves take training, patience, and diligence but deliver amazing results. Practice strengthening your PC muscles whenever you can: at home, in the office, while commuting. The more you practice, the greater the results. Conscientiously practicing these contractions will stimulate what happens naturally during arousal.

The PC muscles are rarely included in most general exercise programs. In yoga, these muscles are activated most directly through "Mula Bundha," literally translated as the sexual energy of the body. To engage the Mula Bundha you'll need to exhale completely. Go ahead, try it now. Then, when your lungs are completely empty, contract your PC muscles and draw in your pelvic floor. You can do this anytime, but it's particularly useful to focus on your Mula Bundha when you are practicing your poses. Ultimately, strengthening those PC muscles can help you achieve explosive orgasms.

Breath and Circulation. We know that the breath and circulation aren't muscles, but these two body functions are important to keeping your love muscles working properly, so we've included them here. Breathing deeply into the abdomen helps the muscles in your sexual core contract and expand, massaging and revitalizing them. Breathe into areas of tightness in order to loosen up, and let your awareness follow your breath. The effect is very subtle at first, but using your breath to develop awareness of your body is a great way to prepare it for lovemaking.

Good circulation has a more direct effect. First, it brings new blood to the area, stimulating and revitalizing the nerves, so that every touch, every movement, and every twist in the bedroom will be felt more deeply and powerfully. Second, it increases your endurance for the physical rigors of sexual activity, to ensure that you'll have tons of enthusiasm and energy for long, luxurious bouts of lovemaking.

The Big O

No discussion about sexual fitness would be complete without mention of the big O: orgasm. Let's face it, we all want longer, better, and more frequent orgasms. So for a moment, let's turn our attention to the East. In eastern mysticism such as yoga, it is believed that the orgasm travels up the body. Starting at the feet, the energy moves through the pelvis (through acupressure points called the "rushing door"), where it gathers pure orgasm energy, then up to the chest, where it mixes with the heart energy, and finally finishing at the face, by encircling the lips and blushing the cheeks. That's the flushed, undeniable glow we get after great sex.

We all know it takes a bit of effort—and skill—for your partner to help you orgasm. Sometimes it works and sometimes it doesn't. That doesn't mean you should take what you get. *Au contraire,* you should do whatever it takes to help yourself get climax-ready too!

Those PC muscles are one of the keys to unlocking the highest level of orgasms. When you orgasm, your PC muscles involuntarily contract, releasing the euphoric sensation of that orgasmic experience. The stronger your PC muscles, the deeper the orgasms, and the easier those orgasms are to achieve.

Another key to achieving explosive orgasms is knowing when to relax your PC muscles during sex. Relaxing them during vaginal stimulation allows for surrender when you are reaching the plateau phase—the moments right before orgasm. Total relaxation through your sexual core allows heightened sensations and invites orgasm to come. Knowing when to relax like this can help you to achieve full-body orgasm; the lucky few can even achieve multiple orgasms.

Did you know you that men can have multiple orgasms? *Better Sex Through Yoga* can help. (Tell your man this right away, and you'll be fighting over this book.) Contracting your PC muscles in a quick, repetitious pattern mimics the effects of multiple orgasms on those muscles. The more you practice, the better chance your man can experience that lengthy rush a multiple orgasm delivers. Often when a man reaches orgasm, he ejaculates sooner than he and his partner would like. More control over those PC muscles and the sexual core can help him sustain an erection *and* last longer before climaxing.

Another way you'll achieve a better orgasm is through the breath. Some of the yoga breathing techniques you'll learn later actually imitate the type of fast breathing that occurs during the peak of the plateau phase and climax of an orgasm. You may want to consider trying the Breath of Fire (page 24) technique to help you stimulate and speed along the plateau phase so that you and your partner have the chance to come together.

And finally, when it comes to achieving orgasm with your partner, remember: You're not in a race! Orgasms are a highlight, an ultimate bonus to sex, but should not be the main goal. They are simply dessert after a very delicious meal.

The Body-Mind-Sex Connection

Your sexual fitness is not just a matter of the physical body being in top shape; your mental and emotional states also play a huge role in your ability to attain sexual fulfillment.

Scientists are learning more and more that emotions are not just "moods." Actually, our emotions represent real physiological states that powerfully impact our physical well-being, including our sexual well-being. It turns out that our mental state can positively or negatively impact all parts of our bodies, from our hearts, to our blood vessels, to our genitals.

So what's the biggest sex-buster? Stress. Our modern, hectic lives are riddled with stress. From the traffic on the roads, to never-ending cell phone calls, to our fast-paced work environments, stress can wreck havoc on our physical health and sexual satisfaction. In fact, *Newsweek* magazine reported that experts now believe that an incredible 60 to 90 percent of all doctor-visits involve stress-related complaints.

Stress can ruin our health and our sex lives, causing us to feel sick and keeping us from sexual activity and fulfillment. But remember that famous old complaint, "Not tonight, dear, I have a headache?" Well, as an educated

Better Sex Through Yoga reader, you know better! Many people avoid sex when they are feeling stressed out; you now know that sex can actually be the *cure* for many stress-related health problems.

Just as negative emotions such as stress can cause us to feel ill, positive emotions can have the opposite effect. Researchers are finding that positive emotions, such as religious faith, optimism, and happiness, can translate into better physical health. Researchers at Harvard University found that prayer, deep-breathing exercises, and, you guessed it, practicing yoga can counteract stress-related health problems.

So you see, it's all interconnected: our physical fitness, our emotional fitness, and our sexual fitness. And the *Better Sex Through Yoga* program is the path to sustaining it all.

Five Keys to Great Sex

Let's take a moment to recap. We don't just want you to have good sex; we want you to have *great* sex. We want you to have the kind of sex our role model Samantha Jones would tell Carrie, Miranda, and Charlotte over brunch. The basis of your sexual fitness comes down to five key areas:

1. SEXUAL CORE
Great sex comes from strong abdominal and pelvic muscles and relaxed hip flexors. Among the most neglected set of muscles in the body, your sexual core muscles are crucial to a more satisfying love life. Healthy PC muscles improve bladder control, encourage more blood flow to the genitals, and enhance sensitivity to both anal and vaginal stimulation.

2. FLEXIBILITY AND STRENGTH
Becoming stronger and more flexible gives you the freedom to have sex longer and more creatively. If your muscles feel tight, they're unnaturally shortened, making anything other than the missionary position feel like work. If you can bend over and touch your palms flat on the ground without passing out during yoga, think of what you'll be able to accomplish during sex.

3. BREATHING

Focused, controlled breathing has the power to defuse anxiety and stress and to boost energy. Breathing exercises facilitate the flow of more oxygen and blood through the entire body, lowering blood pressure, stimulating metabolism, aiding digestion, and releasing the tension around the organs that get in the way of experiencing incredible full-body orgasms. If you learn to breathe calmly and effectively in what seem at first to be some rather awkward, uncomfortable yoga positions, you will be able to stretch out that moment of climax or stay within the moment without fizzling out because of lack of energy or oxygen.

4. BLOOD FLOW

Increased blood flow and circulation in your pelvis not only improves stamina, muscle tone, and sensitivity, it also brings a heightened awareness to the parts of your body involved in sexual response. The blood follows the breath; thus, deep breathing brings more oxygen to your blood, making it rich and full of energy-building potential. Regular practice increases blood flow to the genitals, priming both you and your partner for great sex.

5. MIND-BODY CONNECTION

Our emotions and our mental state are inseparably linked to our physical and sexual well-being. Negative emotions and stress actually can cause and exacerbate physical illness and wreck havoc on our sex lives. Science has shown that yoga can be the key to unlocking the mind-body connection, alleviating stress and reducing stress-related illness. And now you know that sex can contribute to emotional and physical healing as well. Marvin Gaye had it right when he sang about "sexual healing." So let's get started.

3

GETTING STARTED: BETTER SEX THROUGH YOGA BASICS

Before we jump into our *Better Sex Through Yoga* poses and routines (after all this talk about sex and orgasms, we're sure your raring to go), it's important that we cover some basic techniques and concepts that form the foundation for our program. If you're a yoga virgin, you'll need to be especially thorough in practicing all of the basic yoga exercises described in this chapter.

We'll start off with the basics: instructions on breathing, alignment, and what to keep in mind to make your practice—and your sex life—as fantastic as it can be. Then we'll show you some basic yoga techniques that you can try right away and everything you'll need to get started with our program.

Breathe Like a Yogi

We were all born to breathe like yogis. Watch any baby and you'll see that its little belly rises when inhaling and falls when exhaling. The same is true for animals. In fact, each night when you fall asleep, you also revert to this natural and automatic way of breathing. It is the most efficient way of breathing, as it constantly supplies the brain with fresh oxygen. Unfortunately, by the time most of us have reached adulthood, we've forgotten how to breathe this way. At best, we inhale and suck our stomachs in, then exhale and let our bellies expand. Some of us don't move our bellies at all! In all three types of breathing to be discussed, you always inhale and expand your belly, exhale and flatten your belly. Don't worry if you don't master this technique right away. Keep practicing and relearn the yogic way of breathing that will bring you power and potency all day and all night.

Basic Yogic Breathing

Yogic breathing can calm you down or get you pumped up, depending on how you do it. It will help you get centered so you can really experience sex fully. Calm, regular, and deep breathing through the nose gives you an oxygen high, the all-natural buzz that will help bring you to the plateau phase of orgasm and the final release.

TO DO IT Lie flat on your back and relax your legs. Place a hard and slightly heavy (at least one pound) book on your abdomen. Now close your eyes and move your arms to your sides, or place one hand on top of the book. Inhale deeply through your nose, expanding your belly, so the book rises up an inch or two. Then continue to breathe into your lower back, upper abdomen, and chest with your inhale. When you can inhale no more, pause. Then slowly exhale, gently squeezing the air from your chest, upper abdomen, lower back, and finally belly. Notice how the book sank down to its original resting position. Moving the book up and down means that you are successfully breathing deeply into your lower abdomen and not limiting the breath to your chest and shoulders. This is a wonderful way to wind down after a workout, an intense lovemaking session, or anytime you're in need of focus and destressing.

Try this breathing while in different postures. Sit upright in a chair or on the floor. Sit with a straight spine, and keep your shoulders loose. Keep a hand on your abdomen to be sure you are expanding with each inhale. Always breathe in through your nose and down into your belly (which should not be sucked in), then exhale through your nose also.

Use this style of breathing with each and every *Better Sex Through Yoga* pose and routine. When you move with your breath and expand your whole body with each inhale, your yoga practice will be much more effective and enjoyable. In general, faster breathing is more stimulating. For a more restorative and calming effect, make your breaths longer and even deeper.

IN THE BEDROOM Let's face it, during sex it's easy to lose focus and let your mind wander through your daily to-do list. When you start to lose focus in this way, invoke this deep yoga breathing method to keep the moment alive. Breathing at the same rate as your partner will deepen your experience.

BREATH OF FIRE (KAPALABATI BREATHING)
The Breath of Fire method, a series of rapid inhalations and exhalations, is a bit more advanced than basic yogic breathing. Its purpose is to rid your lungs of stale air and open the way for fresh, new air to energize your whole body and tone up your abdomen.

TO DO IT Kneel with your butt on your heels, and place your hands on your knees. Inhale through your mouth, drawing your breath down to your lower belly, and allow your abdomen to balloon out as it expands with air. Then exhale sharply through your mouth as if you're trying to shush a talker in a movie theater.

As you blow out, contract your stomach inward and push the air outward, then inhale and allow your belly to expand, creating a vacuum that brings air back in. Allow your body to naturally take in this next breath, and breathe out hard again while your abdomen expands and contracts with each cycle. Be sure to inhale and exhale fully during each cycle. Do not allow for one inhale to last for several exhales! Do thirty breaths for your first set at about one breath per second. On your second set, do sixty counts and double the pace, to closer to two breaths per second. Attractive, we know. But it'll give you a ton of energy and expel stress, which is key for great sex.

If you're having trouble, lay a hand on your belly to be sure it moves in and out. Place the index finger of your other hand in front of your mouth to help you feel your breath. Keep your back straight and your shoulders relaxed and away from your ears. Try to isolate the pumping action in your abdomen without raising your shoulders each time. Remember, every time your stomach goes in and out, you're tightening your sexual core a little more.

IN THE BEDROOM During sex, Breath of Fire is especially useful for intensifying the climax phase of orgasm, once you've reached the point of no return and orgasm is imminent. This technique is particularly useful if you take longer to reach orgasm than your partner. If you notice that your partner is beginning to pant faster and you want to move along to keep at his pace, invoke the Breath of Fire to fast-forward your pleasure. This invigorating style of yogic breathing boosts circulation and increases oxygen to internal organs, which elevates desire. It also strengthens the abs and contracts the muscles in the sexual core.

THREE-PART BREATH

Calming and rejuvenative, this breathing style will restore your body's natural healing responses. What's more, it helps to build energy: sexually, physically, and mentally. Three-Part Breathing works best when lying down in a quiet place, and is enhanced by the use of an eye pillow (a silk sack filled with herbs or seeds that soothes the eyes) or by dimming the lights and closing your eyes.

TO DO IT Lie on your back. Inhale through your nose, and breathe into your sexual core, below your belly button and into your abdomen. Then, while keeping your sexual core expanded, keep inhaling and fill your chest with air, so that your lungs and chest swell. Finally, while maintaining the expanse in your sexual core and in your chest, bring your breath to your lower throat, that sexy place where your collarbone meets your neck. Pause here briefly, then exhale through your nose in reverse by emptying your throat first, then your chest, and, finally, your sexual core or lower belly. Repeat ten times slowly. Take your time, and breathe in and out as deeply as you can—ideally counting to six as you inhale, pausing for a count, and then exhaling for eight counts.

IN THE BEDROOM Try this while experiencing the excitement phase (foreplay) or plateau phase (mounting sexual tension), right before the Breath of Fire, for a mind-blowing orgasm. For those of you who are in need of a little bedroom TLC, using this breathing style will recalibrate your nervous system. In particular, Three-Part Breath can help you to deepen your connection with your lover. By breathing slowly and synchronizing your breath, you and your partner can begin to experience emotions of the heart such as giving, receiving, sharing, and deep unconditional love.

Stand Like a Yogi

Proper alignment is crucial in yoga. The backbone—if you will—of proper alignment is ultimately your posture. Sadly, good posture is not something all of us are born with. And because so many of us sit for prolonged hours at our jobs, on our commute, and on the couch when we finally get home at the end of the day, it's also something that many of us ignore. Correcting years of bad posture takes time, but with our instructions and some focused work on your part, you can begin to reverse this.

Your posture says a lot about you. It can say "I am confident, happy and open to giving and receiving love," or it can say just the opposite. Good posture builds self-empowerment, lets you look better in (and out of) your clothes, and gives you an air of confidence; bad posture gives off the impression that you are shrinking away from the world or are tired and withdrawn.

How does all of this relate to hotter sex? Proper alignment of your body in yoga, as in sex, will help to ensure a more graceful and effective performance while allowing your body's energy and blood flow to move freely and abundantly. To help you focus on your body alignment, we've designed two simple exercises that you can do practically anywhere, anytime. Mastering these techniques will help you on the mat *and* in the bedroom.

Perfect Alignment while Seated

This exercise supports your lower back and prevents chronic back pain, as well as low sexual energy—it also develops gorgeous abdominal muscles all day long!

TO DO IT Start by placing both feet flat on the floor. Squat down and keep your thighs parallel to the floor. If your knees and hips are not level, place a phone book under your feet. Your weight should be centered over your pelvic bones, and your head should be balanced directly in between your shoulders. Elongate the back of your neck by slightly tucking your chin toward your chest. Always engage your abdominal muscles by pulling your navel toward your spine. When you inhale, allow your abdomen to balloon out slightly; when you exhale, contract your abdominal muscles to expel your breath. Always keep your shoulders low and away from your ears and your chest open and pointing forward.

IN THE BEDROOM Having a strong seated posture will help with many sex positions, including the Rearview, Yin Yang, and Rock Steady. (Take a sneak peek at our hot sex positions in Chapter 7.)

PERFECT ALIGNMENT WHILE STANDING

This exercise promotes the natural curve in your lower back and keeps your head centered on top of your spine.

TO DO IT Stand with your feet a few inches apart and your toes spread. Distribute your weight evenly on your feet; don't lean back on your heels or roll to the sides of your feet. Point your toes and knees forward using the muscles that surround your knees. Don't lock your knees; instead, keep them slightly bent, with the thigh muscles firm and lifting upward.

Next, lengthen the space between your navel and your collarbone by lifting your collarbone up toward the ceiling. Align your shoulders under your ears, and let your arms hang gracefully at your sides with a slight bend to the elbow, palms facing your thighs. As mentioned in the "Basic Yogic Breathing" instructions, breathe into your entire chest and abdomen, including the lower back. Inhale and expand with your breath, exhale and squeeze the air up and out with your abdominal strength.

IN THE BEDROOM What better way to excite your partner than with a pre-sex peep show? Standing like a yogi when donning that next-to-nothing nightie will make him hot!

Making Sense of Your Chakras

Does being flexible, generous, loving, satisfied, and balanced sound like the way you'd like to be in your relationship? Doing *Better Sex Through Yoga* regularly will build up these characteristics within you because, aside from all of the physical benefits we've been raving about, practicing yoga brings balance to the energy flow through your body and awakens your sexual energy. This energy flow is cultivated and housed in your chakras, and you'll soon understand why chakras are so important to the *Better Sex Through Yoga* program.

First some chakra basics. *Chakra* is a Sanskrit word meaning "vortex" or "energy center." Like acupressure points, chakras function like little valves that regulate the flow of chi (the energy source throughout your body). Depending on your actions and thoughts, chakras open and close, shaping perceptions and experiences. Due to under- or overexercising, prolonged sitting or poor eating habits, your chakras can become blocked. Emotional issues can also block your chakras, resulting in feelings of depression, low self-esteem, jealousy, and possessiveness.

Yoga can keep your chakras unclogged and clear so that you can feel true satisfaction and love for yourself and your partner. When you turn that focus toward your sexual practice, you'll experience sex and consciousness at a whole new level.

Better Sex Through Yoga helps to unlock the seven major chakras, giving you an idea of which of your chakras may be out of balance and what yoga moves you can do to revamp them. As you read through the descriptions of each chakra, physically locate each one on your body and gently massage the area. (Hint: You may want to do this in private.) Once you've found your own chakras, we encourage you to place your hands on and gently massage your partner's chakras during sex. This should feel pleasurable, satisfying, and comforting to you both.

The Seven Major Chakras

First Chakra. This chakra is located at the lower spine. When the first chakra is out of balance, your sense of safety is threatened, and you could have difficulty expressing yourself in a free, creative, and flexible way. In relationships, having the first chakra out of balance can hinder your ability to give and receive unrestrained, passionate love. This chakra may be the culprit if you are possessive, both with time and possessions, and unable to openly share with your lover. You could call it being a "tight-ass," which, given the location of this chakra, can be very true! Keep yourself flexible and loose

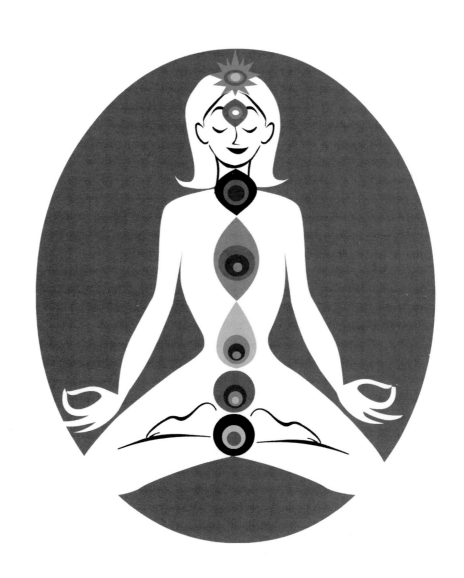

while practicing generosity with your sweetie, and this chakra will be in better balance and will improve your sex life and your relationship overall.

Second Chakra. The famed "sex chakra" located in the genital region, the second chakra is the seat of grace, depth of feeling, creativity, and sexual fulfillment for both sexes. It is also the chakra most in need of more attention, love, and acceptance so that we may experience intimacy and closeness during lovemaking. When properly balanced, this chakra enhances sex drive, reproduction, and animal magnetism. Conversely, when it is out of balance, sexual difficulties, emotional instability, dissatisfaction, frustration, and preoccupation with your physical appearance will surface. If you keep fluidity, relaxation, and pleasure in mind when you make love or do yoga, you will find that this chakra gets very happy.

Third Chakra. The third chakra is located in the lower abdomen and governs metabolism and digestion. The overall energy production and storage center of the body, it is easy for this area to go out of whack with overconsumption of food or alcohol. A blockage in this energy center causes the energy needed for digestion, metabolism, gut feelings, self-esteem, and confidence to stagnate. To better help your love life and cultivate self-love, be up front with your emotions, follow your instincts, and do not overeat. Also, be sure to practice yogic breathing so that you develop lean, beautiful abdominal muscles, which help to keep this area in harmony.

Fourth Chakra. Known as the heart chakra, this energy center is located in the center of the chest, directly at heart level. The heart chakra's mantra could be: Open yourself to love and realize that the more you love, the easier it is to give and receive love. A healthy heart chakra encourages you to feel compassion, love deeply, be devoted, and feel at peace. You can avoid being needy, depressed, and fearful of rejection in your relationships by doing the appropriate yoga poses to clear the fourth chakra. Practice sitting with perfect posture to prevent collapsed shoulders and an inhibited heart.

Fifth Chakra. The key center for communication, the fifth chakra is located in the throat. This chakra governs finding your voice, whether through dancing, painting, singing, or moaning in ecstasy when aroused. Since communication is vital for a successful sexual relationship, strengthening this chakra is a must. Tell your partner what you want and vocalize what you need to maintain and build your identity. Truth and self-expression are musts. Your relationship will flourish when you balance this chakra by speaking straight from your heart.

Sixth Chakra. Insight, vision, and imagination are just a few of the qualities associated with the sixth chakra. Located in between your eyebrows, this psychic center is often referred to as the third eye. This chakra also governs having clarity about your identity, your sexual being, and your "self" as seen by others. Bringing stability to this energy center will help you to see yourself as others do, so that you can make changes to correct unsavory behavior. Poor memory, balance, and concentration are all signs of a blocked third eye. Some of the balancing poses in Chapter 4 help to unlock this chakra.

Seventh Chakra. Located at the very top (or crown) of your head, the seventh chakra is the pivotal point for higher consciousness, bliss, and spiritual connection. Your ability to maintain relationships and sense that you are truly understood relate to this chakra. When you and your partner are able to reach this heightened state of consciousness together while making love, your orgasms will be blissful and mind-blowing.

Strike a Pose

Yoga is made up of over two hundred poses, or *asansas,* and each pose works your body in its own distinct way. In this book, we've taken some of those poses and put our own sexual twist on them. Some poses may be familiar if you've practiced yoga before; others we've modified to help bring out the sexual vixen in you.

For each pose, make sure to maintain good posture and move with grace and precision. Try to use powerful deep breathing rather than loud grunts or groans if you're finding a pose particularly challenging. Your breath will give you added strength. Never just "hang out" in a pose; rather, keep extending, lifting, and reaching throughout the entire pose as you breathe. And be sure to keep your face and jaw muscles soft and relaxed; this will stop you from straining unnecessarily (a slight smile will naturally prevent this).

To keep things simple, we've grouped our yoga poses into five categories:

Warm-up and Transition. The warm-up and transition moves help energize and heat up your body. The Sun Salutation and Basic Beauty are two corner-stones of all *Better Sex Through Yoga* routines. During the routines you will be cued to do several Sun Salutations. This is also a series of postures linked together, rather than one stand-alone pose, and it is important that you learn how to do it properly before you tackle anything more advanced. The most important thing to focus on when practicing these moves is linking your movement to your breath, carefully follow the breath cues as you practice. The Basic Beauty, our special *Better Sex Through Yoga* warm-up flow, takes about five minutes to complete. It gently stretches the neck, hamstrings, and lower back before you begin doing yoga, so that you'll be loose and open.

Duo Assisted Poses. Massaging tight spots, full-body contact, and gently coaxing your partner's tight areas to loosen them makes practicing yoga even more fun. These Duo Assisted poses will help you to push the limits of your comfort zone. Assisting your lover with these poses is not only great sensual foreplay, but also a great way to focus on your physical and emotional communication. Becoming more sexually fit together demonstrates your commitment to each other and to your sexual desires.

Floor Poses. Since many sexual positions are performed in a lying-down position, the poses we've selected really pinpoint the areas that need the most attention in the bedroom. The relaxation poses, including Chill Out (page 60), are just as important as the more strenuous, such as Camel (page 62) and Crane (page 58).

Standing Poses. The standing poses are a diverse mix of poses that build balance, strength, and flexibility. When you perform these poses, you really want to focus on centering your body and feeling grounded. The intense focus you'll need for many of these standing poses will help you focus your sexual energy too.

Sexy Secretary Poses. Since we're already multitasking, you might as well take your yoga practice to the office chair so you can feel sexy 24/7. Prolonged sitting often is the cause of dulled nerve endings, bad posture, and a dampened sex life. Keeping a perfect posture all day at work is a huge workout that will engage muscles throughout the entire body, burning calories as well as toning your deep inner sexual core muscles. Incorporate these poses into your workday to fight fatigue, help prevent bloating, and most of all, keep sexy.

The Better Sex Through Yoga Poses

In the next chapters, we've broken down each pose using the same formula, so that you can get the most out of each and every *Better Sex Through Yoga* pose. We suggest reading through the entire explanation first before giving it a try on the mat. Here's what you'll find.

POSITION NAME For some of the poses, we've kept the traditional yoga names (like Downward Dog); for others (like Cupid's Arrow), we've sexed up the titles to help get you in the mood. In this section, you'll also find a brief explanation of how each pose will benefit your body, mind, and spirit (and, oh yes, your sex life).

TO DO IT This is the heart of the explanation. Here you'll find detailed instructions to get in and out of the pose as well as precise photos to help you visualize the pose. You'll also find important breathing cues.

VARIATIONS Once you've mastered the basic pose, we've added some intermediate and advanced poses that help build on the basic pose and will help you add variation to your routine.

CHAKRAS Each pose affects your energy flow—and your emotions—in different ways. We've listed which chakras come into play for each pose.

HOTTIE BODY Looking to sculpt that "hottie" yoga butt of yours? Here we've pinpointed which major body parts will benefit from each pose.

IN THE BEDROOM We like this category the best and hope you will too. Here we've identified which sexual positions mimic the principles and positions in each particular pose. In Chapter 7, "Mind-Blowing Sex Positions," you'll find a complete list of all of these positions. Go ahead, take a sneak peek now. See what your reward is for all the work you'll do.

hot tip **{** Finally, we offer you a hot tip to help you achieve maximum sexual results from the pose and get you, well, hot and in the mood for sex.

The Better Sex Through Yoga Routines

Once you're familiar with all of the basic poses in Chapter 4, you'll be ready to put those poses together into sequences we call the *Better Sex Through Yoga* Routines. Going from one pose to the next in yoga is called a "flow." Flows are a sequence of postures or movements linked together through your breath. There are a few types of routines you'll need to know about.

Core Routines. The core routines are the basic building blocks of the *Better Sex Through Yoga* program. Each routine is made up of a variety of poses and as well as warm-up and transition moves, and we've designed each one for specific results in the bedroom. These routines are all about flow, so always focus on linking your breath to the movement. Ultimately, as your body becomes stronger, your breath deeper, and your mind more focused, you will be able to flow through all the routines more easily and with greater grace.

Quickie Routines. Similar to the core routines, the quickie routines are designed to give you quick stimulation and quick results. It's like a quick fix before sex. (Though obviously we don't want the sex to be quick!)

Practice Makes Puuurfect

Once you're familiar with all of the *Better Sex Through Yoga* poses and warm-up and transition moves, you'll be ready to move on to the core routines. Start off by doing one routine of your choice three times each week. You can supplement the core routines with some quickies too. Or you can do the quickies when the right mood hits you.

The routines will prepare your body physically for great sex, but they are also designed with flow, groove, and rhythm. To sync up with the mood, you still need a psychological cue. Desire, confidence, and lust come from your mind. Use your imagination. Set your mind to feeling more sexually engaged and powerful, and it will happen.

Before You Begin

Once you've set the mood and created your own private space for practicing *Better Sex Through Yoga*, here are some other things to keep in mind as you embark on your journey to better sex:

- Consult your doctor before beginning *Better Sex Through Yoga*. If you are pregnant or trying to conceive then do not perform any of the exercises in this book.
- Do not eat a big meal at least four hours before doing yoga. Proper breathing and posture are hard to maintain when your belly is full.
- Do not wear shoes or socks. You should always practice yoga in bare feet.
- Wear comfortable clothing that can move with you. (If you want to feel really sultry, or you're doing a routine with a partner, wear as little as possible!)
- Practice on a nonskid surface, such as a hardwood floor. A sticky yoga mat is best, and you can buy one just about anywhere these days. A few poses call for a chair. Any hard chair you have around

the house is fine; just make sure it's resting on a flat, hard surface and won't slip and slide around.

- Trust your body. You should feel challenged and engaged while doing these poses, but if something hurts or just feels wrong, stop doing it. There's no need to push yourself beyond your own comfort level.

- Last, remember why you are doing this. Stay focused on your goal to look and feel sexier, be more full of love, and find more sexual satisfaction.

Now set the mood by dimming the lights, closing the windows, and adjusting the temperature to "warm." Pop in your favorite CD, light some candles, and get going.

4

BETTER SEX THROUGH YOGA BASIC POSES

WARM-UPS AND TRANSITIONS

There are two moves that you'll be doing quite a bit throughout our program—Sun Salutation and Basic Beauty—which are actually a series of moves linked together by your breath. Sometimes we'll use these moves as warm-ups at the beginning of a routine to get the blood flowing and body and breath ready. You may even want to give these moves a try before sex. When we say "blood flowing," we mean *everywhere*—including the parts that matter most during sex, like your brain. (You've probably heard that your brain is your biggest sexual organ, so we want blood to flow there too.) Other times we'll use these moves as transitions within a routine to go from one pose to the next. Either way, these moves are an important part of our program. If you're new to yoga, you may want to read through all of the instructions first, then look at the detailed explanations of the poses later on in the chapter.

SUN SALUTATION

Throughout the Better Sex Through Yoga *routines, except for one or two, you will be instructed to do a Sun Salutation preceding a position, or group of positions. On the routine pages, you will see the Sun Salutation used quite often. So what exactly is a Sun Salutation? In Hindu mythology, the Sun Salutation originated as a series of worship to the sun. The sequence of poses is traditionally performed early in the morning, as the sun rises. A graceful flow of positions threaded one after another and done in combination with the breath, the Sun Salutation limbers up the body in preparation for the posture to follow. When combined with cued breathing, the Sun Salutation is a continuous exercise that alternatively stretches, expands, and contracts the whole body, working all major muscle groups while massaging the internal organs. It also gets the blood flowing and shakes up those sex muscles. As always, deep, rhythmic breathing is a must, but how fast you breathe will determine how fast you will move through the routine. Remember, move faster for a more stimulating and vigorous workout and move slower for a more restorative and calming workout. Either way, you will finish feeling refreshed, balanced, and, we hope, more joyful and loving.*

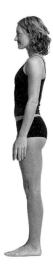

TO DO IT Begin by standing with your feet together, arms at your side.

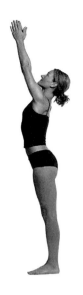

Next, inhale, raise both arms above your head, touch your palms together, and look toward the sky.

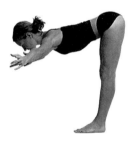

Exhale, and dive forward with a flat back and your chin lifted.

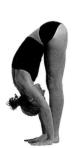

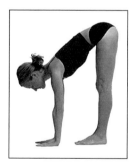

Place your hands on the floor next to your feet, with your head facing your shins. If you can't reach the ground, try extending your hands forward until you can do so while contracting your stomach to pelvic muscles (see inset).

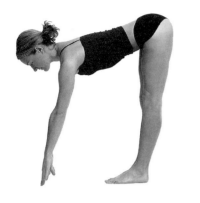

Inhale and lift your hands onto your fingertips, keeping your back flat and your chest lifted. Look forward.

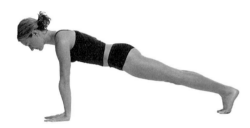

Exhale, place your hands back on the ground, and step back one foot at a time into the Plank (page 44). Gaze between your hands with your arms straight, keeping your stomach flat and your body straight like a board. (This is a long exhale, so conserve your breath.)

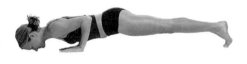

Keep exhaling, and bend your arms, lowering to the bottom of a push-up. Keep your elbows at your sides with your back straight, and touch your nose to the floor.

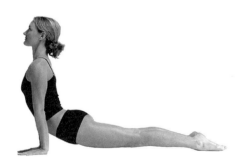

Inhale and push up and into the Upward Dog (page 48). Your back should be arched, with your arms straight at your sides. Lift your hip bones off the floor and lower your shoulders away from your ears. Gaze straight ahead with your feet pointed, weight placed on the top of your feet on the floor. Keep your legs squeezed tight and muscular.

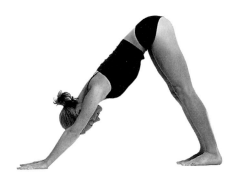

Exhale, curl your toes under, and press the soles of your feet to the floor while you lift your pelvis up and into the Downward Dog (page 130).

Tilt your pelvis forward with your tailbone facing the ceiling. Flex your feet and lower your heels toward the ground, elongating your neck by gazing above your kneecaps. Press your hands flat onto the floor with your fingers spread out. Hold for five full body breaths.

BASIC BEAUTY

This series of postures is one of the best ways to welcome the day, get ready for a hot date, or chill out before a big event. It unkinks the muscles in your back as well as the long muscles along the front and backs of your legs and the pesky knotted muscles around your neck.

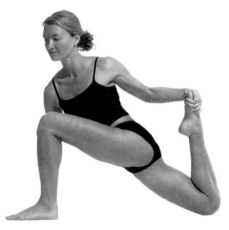

TO DO IT

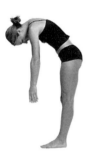

With your feet hip distance apart, lower your head and shoulders forward and roll toward the floor. Touch your hands to the floor, bending your knees if necessary, and relax your neck, gazing between your legs. First nod your head up and down yes, then shake your head side to side no.

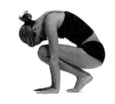

Bend down into a squat, tuck your chin to your chest, and pulse your hips and knees in a small bounce. Straighten your legs and stand again in a forward bend while looking behind you, between your legs. Bend, squat, and pulse twice more.

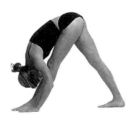

Step your right leg back about three feet and stand with your legs separate and your forehead toward your front shin. Relax your shoulders and neck, and keep both legs straight. If necessary, bend your back knee only, but keep your front leg straight. Hold for four breaths.

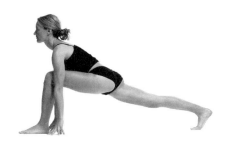

Step your right leg back even farther and lower into a lunge with your front knee bent, your back heel reaching behind you. Look straight ahead and hold for four breaths. Then lower your back knee, rest the top of your foot on the floor, and tuck your chin to your chest. Hold for two breaths.

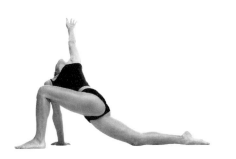

Lower your right palm to the floor, and reach your left arm high up toward the ceiling. Look up at your hand, then reach your arm farther over your back and gently twist your back. Hold for two breaths. (Basically you are doing a spinal twist while kneeling.)

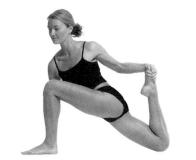

Circle your left arm behind you, bend your right knee, and hold the top of your right foot, pulling it toward your tail-bone. (This is a fantastic quadriceps stretch.) Hold for two breaths.

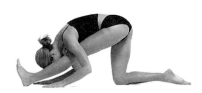

Straighten out your left leg and flex your foot, with your toes toward the ceiling. While kneeling on your right knee, bend at the waist, keeping your back flat and lowering your head toward your left knee. Hold for two deep breaths.

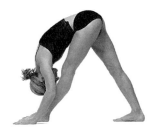

Rise, straighten, and separate your legs. Keep your head toward your shin. Turn all the way around and face the opposite side of the room, with your right leg in front now, and repeat the entire flow on this side.

43

FLOOR POSES

Whether you're sitting, lying, twisting, or bending, all of these floor poses focus on centering your body through your pelvis. And as we mentioned before, the pelvis is one of the key areas to developing your sexual core. Don't be afraid to use your imagination and visualize yourself intertwined with your partner during these poses. Let your imagination run wild and feel your pelvis and sexual core flow with excitement as you try the Locust (page 66) and Pelvic Squeezes (page 84). Then let all that sexual energy release with some of the relaxation poses, such as At Peace (page 128) and Easy Spinal Twist (page 124).

PLANK
This move builds shoulder strength, lengthens the spine, and strengthens the lower back muscles while toning the abdomen and sexual core. It also appears in Chapter 7 as Surf's Up.

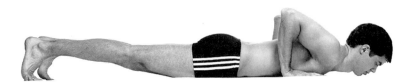

TO DO IT Lie down with your chin on the floor. Look forward slightly and encourage the natural cervical curve behind your neck. Place your thumbs underneath your nipples, fingers facing forward and spread wide.

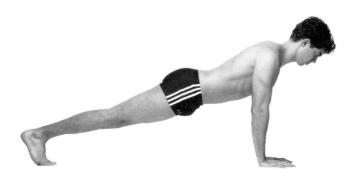

Keep your elbows close by your side, tuck your toes under, and rise to your balls of your feet. Push your heels back and flex the back of your legs, knees off the floor. Align your hips so your tailbone is pointing toward your feet and your lower back is straight. Inhale deeply, then exhale, hold your body tight, and straighten your arms into a perfect plank.

CHAKRAS 2, 3

HOTTIE BODY	• tight triceps
	• gorgeous biceps
	• yummy tummy

IN THE BEDROOM	• Bundled Package
	• The Conquest
	• Surf's Up

hot tip { Make sure to keep your whole body hard but your face relaxed. When you practice this pose, try to imagine lowering yourself up and down (and up and down . . .) over your partner using your new strong arms.

PLANK POSE SIDE

This pose tones your obliques and abdomen while challenging your balance. Resist the urge to "muscle" your way through this pose. Instead, practice feeling your body very light.

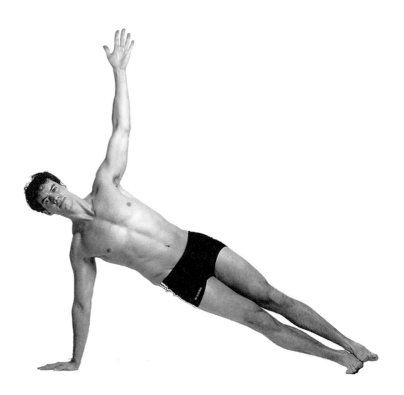

TO DO IT From Plank (page 44), place your right palm underneath your chin. Move your right foot a couple of inches toward the center of your mat, in line with your right palm. Rotate your body toward the left, balancing on the outside of your right foot and right hand. Your heels should be touching, legs straight, and feet flexed. Lift your hips up so that you make a straight line from underneath your left armpit to the edge of your left heel. Reach your left arm toward the ceiling, making both arms one straight line. Make sure to reach up continuously toward the left hand so you do not collapse into your right shoulder. Look down at your right hand, and keep your neck in line with your spine. Breathe in and out into your sexual core five times. To release, bring your left hand down to the floor and return to Plank. Repeat on the other side.

CHAKRAS 3, 4

HOTTIE BODY
- strong obliques
- sculpted lats
- sexy shoulders

IN THE BEDROOM
- Bathing Beauties
- Bridging the Gap
- Surf's Up
- Wild Child

hot tip { Keep your abs and obliques firm and your neck and face relaxed. Make sure your body is in one straight line and that your hips don't sag. Then try this pose face to face with your lover. Can you hold the pose still enough so that you can French kiss?

UPWARD DOG

This pose is an excellent fatigue fighter. It strengthens your spine, arms, and wrists while aligning your spine and improving your posture. You'll also feel increased blood flow in your sexual core, and firmer butt and calf muscles.

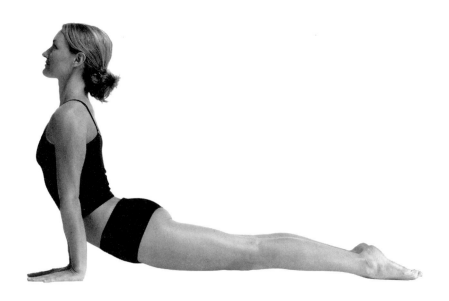

TO DO IT Begin in Plank (page 44). Exhale and lower down to one inch off the floor. Inhale, drop your shoulders down and back, slide your body forward and press your chest forward, and stretch the crown of your head up toward the ceiling. At the same time, lift your thighs and legs off the floor by pressing the tops of your feet into the floor. Keep your legs taut all the way up to your sexual core, and keep your butt firm but not too hard. Breathe in and out five times. To release, put the balls of your feet into the floor, exhale, and lift your hips into Downward Dog (page 130).

CHAKRAS 2, 4, 7

HOTTIE BODY
- yoga butt
- yummy tummy
- tight triceps
- sculpted lats
- defined calves

IN THE BEDROOM
- Orgasmic Camel
- The Conquest
- Doggie Style
- Oops, I Dropped the Soap!

hot tip { Keep your shoulders down and away from your ears, and press your chest forward. Beginners, if at first you can't raise yourself off your legs, that's okay. Try to keep your legs straight and arch your back only slightly, being sure not to pinch your lower back. This is also an amazing move to try while in Doggie Style. Stretch your legs, arch your back, and enjoy.

ON ALL FOURS

This is a starting point and principal pose for understanding how Better Sex Through Yoga *works. Used in many of the floor postures, On All Fours helps lengthen and realign the spine. Mastering the subtleties of this pelvic tilt will help you find the perfect angle for achieving explosive orgasms. Feeling the effects of tilting your pelvis forward and backward will make all the difference, both in your yoga practice and your sexual satisfaction.*

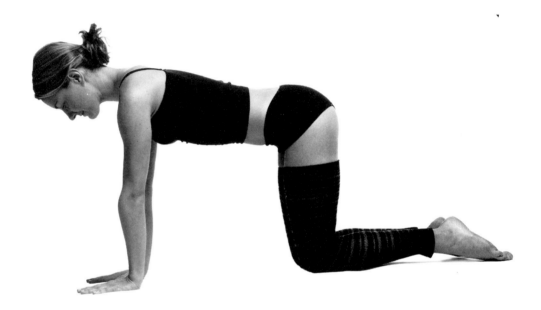

TO DO IT This pose is just like it sounds: Get on all fours. Your knees should be a hip's width apart with your feet lined up directly behind your knees. Place your hands directly under your shoulders with your fingers facing forward and spread out wide. Look down between your palms and keep your back neutral and relaxed. (By "neutral," we mean to allow your back's natural lumbar curve to be present. Do not arch your back or overcontract your abdomen.) Make the back of your neck long and reach the crown of your head toward the front wall. Support your spine by slightly contracting your abs, elongating your back and keeping your hips loose. Don't let your back droop down and sag.

HOTTIE BODY
- loose hips
- flexible lower back
- pliable pelvis

IN THE BEDROOM
- Doggie Style
- Erotic Froggie
- Oops, I Dropped the Soap!

hot tip { Remember, this is a "neutral" pose. This means that you should feel subtle lifting and aligning rather than any type of straining. These subtle movements in the pelvis will lead to explosive orgasms.

SEX KITTEN

This aptly named pose opens the pelvis and lengthens and strengthens the abs and back. This move is a total turn-on for those doing it—and for those watching too! But most important, it stimulates the body's natural flow of sexual and reproductive energy that runs up the front of the body and down the back.

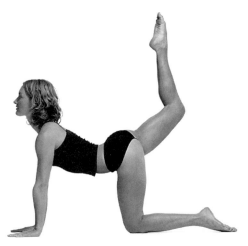

TO DO IT

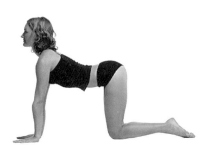

Begin in On All Fours (page 50), looking at the floor between your hands. Your back should be in a neutral and rested state. Keep your butt directly over your knees. Inhale, tilt your pelvis forward with your tailbone up, and arch your back. Look straight ahead.

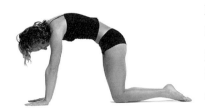

Exhale, tilt your pelvis back, and tuck your tailbone under. Bring your chin to your chest and look at your belly button, pressing the middle of your spine up toward the ceiling, as if trying to touch your spine with your belly button. Repeat eight times, breathing in and out of your sexual core.

VARIATION

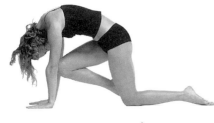

Begin in On All Fours, then shift your weight to your left knee, exhale, and bend your right knee in toward your nose, keeping your toes pointed. Then inhale and raise your leg up as high as you can, pause, and arch your back.

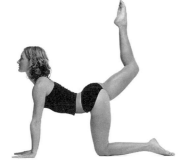

Lower your leg, and again bring your knee to your nose as you exhale. Repeat eight times on each side.

CHAKRAS 1 to 7

HOTTIE BODY
· yoga butt
· yummy tummy
· supple back
· relaxed neck

IN THE BEDROOM
· Orgasmic Camel
· Doggie Style
· Double Triangle
· Erotic Froggie

hot tip { Move into a full back bend each time; don't just isolate your lower back. Keep your fingers splayed and your palms pressing into the floor. Have your man enter you from behind, and do the Sex Kitten move for an extra-hot turn-on.

CHASING TAIL *A sexy, light twist that defines the waist-line, this move also stretches out your hips, butt, and back, increases circulation, and makes it easier to look your lover in the eye while in Doggie Style.*

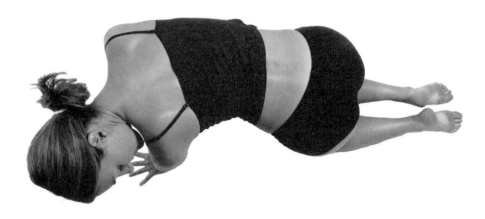

TO DO IT Start in On All Fours (page 50). Bend your hips over to the right side, seriously curving your waist, and look over your right shoulder, as if you're going to see your tail (see inset). Keep your hips parallel to the floor and breathe in and out once, then shift to the other side. Repeat eight times.

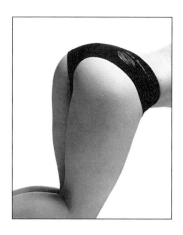

CHAKRAS 1, 3

**HOTTIE
BODY**
· whittled waistline
· yoga butt
· flexible back
· toned thighs

**IN THE
BEDROOM**
· Doggie Style
· Oops, I Dropped the Soap!
· Rearview
· Satisfying Side

hot tip { Keep your tailbone pointing back so your stomach stays firm. For best results, alternate between this move and Sex Kitten while your lover enters you from behind. The side-to-side friction is unbelievable.

FROGGIE

This pose opens and stretches the hips, groin, and inner thighs. It also is the basis for the Erotic Froggie, making it a good one to master.

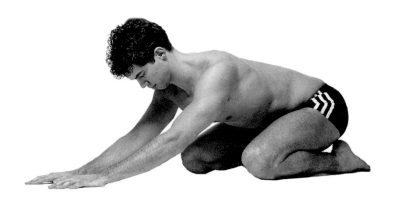

TO DO IT Starting on your knees, lower to your forearms and slide your knees out to the side. Bring your ankles directly in between your knees with the soles of your feet facing each other or touching. Keep your hip bones on the floor, and reach your tailbone toward your feet.

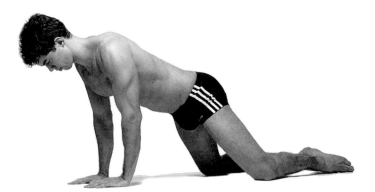

Come forward supporting your torso weight on your arms. Press your feet into the floor, spreading your knees wide.

Lower your torso to the floor as you extend your arms forward. Press your hips down as you lower your ankles to the floor (see inset). It's okay if your feet don't touch the floor; over time they will. Breathe in and out of your sexual core five times.

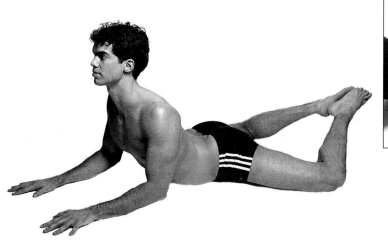

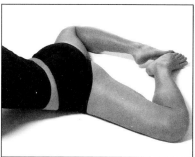

CHAKRAS 1, 2

HOTTIE BODY
- killer inner thighs
- yoga butt
- open hips
- pliable pelvis

IN THE BEDROOM
- Doggie Style
- Erotic Froggie
- Yin Yang

hot tip { When you become really flexible from practicing this pose, use this delicious pose to experience any sex positions from the rear. It's a very flattering position for your mate to see you in.

CRANE
A deep strengthener of your inner sexual core, this position also firms your arms, wrists, and shoulders while opening and toning your groin and abdominal organs.

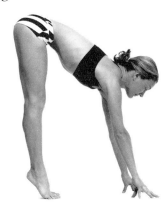

TO DO IT Bend over and reach your arms out in front of you. Raise your heels off the floor, squeeze in your sexual core, and walk forward a few inches.

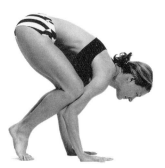

Place your palms flat on the floor in front of you, a bit wider than shoulder-width apart, with your fingers spread. Squat down with your feet hip-width apart and bring your knees behind your elbows. Bend your elbows slightly into your body, rest your knees against your triceps or upper arms, and keep the balls of your feet on the ground with your heels up high. This is an excellent position to build the sexual core by using the abdominal muscle group to keep your tailbone lifted, drawing weight off your arms. Focus on a point in front of you. Tighten your abs downward into your sexual core; you should feel as if you could use them to lift your legs and butt toward the ceiling.

Breathe in and out of your sexual core five times, then release the position. If you feel as if you are about to pitch forward, you're on the right track. Hold the pose as long as you can—even if for only a second. Keep practicing, as the pose will get easier.

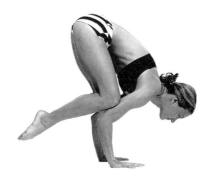

VARIATION Lean your entire body's weight forward onto the back of your upper arms (your triceps), keeping your feet off the floor. Perch in this position by contracting the front of your torso while completely rounding out your back. Lean your body toward your focal point and try to straighten your elbows as far as they will go. Hold where comfortable, and breathe in and out of your sexual core five times. To release, lower your feet to the floor.

CHAKRAS 1, 2, 3

HOTTIE BODY
- yummy tummy
- sexy upper arms

IN THE BEDROOM
- Backseat Buddies
- Bathing Beauties
- Rearview
- Talking in Tongues

hot tip { Have you ever fantasized about having impromptu sex in a small space, like the backseat of a car? Practicing this pose will help make those tight squeezes easier to manage.

CHILL OUT

This pose stretches the lower back, massages your abdominal organs, and stimulates digestion. A counterpose to strenuous back bends and an excellent resting spot if you ever feel exhausted or dizzy, this is the ultimate chill-out pose.

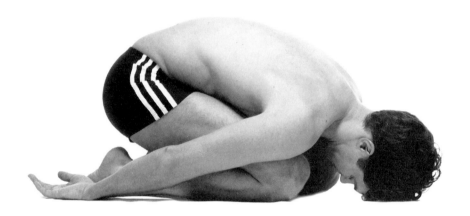

TO DO IT Starting in On All Fours (page 50), lower your butt to your heels and place your forehead on the floor. You can stretch your arms overhead with your palms on the floor, or you can place them alongside your body with your palms toward the ceiling. Breathe deeply, expanding your lower back, then exhale, actively pressing your stomach against your thighs. Repeat five times. To release, place your palms under your shoulders, inhale, and slowly push up to a seated position, on your heels.

CHAKRAS 2, 3, 6

HOTTIE BODY
- beautiful face
- loose hips
- flexible lower back

IN THE BEDROOM
- Bundled Package
- Erotic Froggie
- Wild Child

hot tip { This is a great pose to do after a long day to help you calm down and get in the mood for sex. Chilling out is just the thing to get your mind off your to-do list and onto sex. Take a few minutes to chill and unwind before sex.

CAMEL

This move promotes full back flexibility, stretches the tops of your thighs and pelvis, and opens the heart. It is also the base of our Orgasmic Camel sex position you'll see at the end of the book.

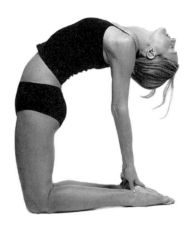

TO DO IT

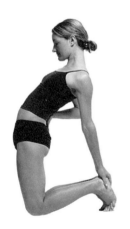

Kneeling on the floor, open your knees slightly wider than your hips. Flex your feet so that the balls of the feet touch the floor.

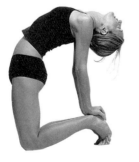

Place your hands on your lower back, squeeze your butt tight, and press your hips forward. Tuck your chin to your chest and then, slowly and gently, reach one hand at a time back and wrap your hands around your heels. Arch your back into a full back bend, as if bending backward over a barrel. If possible, release your head backward, open your chest toward the ceiling, and relax your throat. Take five deep breaths.

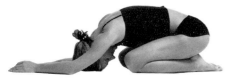

After you release, be sure to chill out for a moment with your head on the floor to realign your blood flow.

VARIATION When your flexibility improves, lower the tops of your feet to the floor.

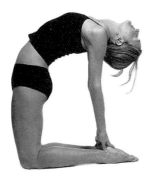

CHAKRAS 2, 3, 4

HOTTIE BODY
- long, lean thighs
- loose hips
- open chest

IN THE BEDROOM
- Doggie Style
- Orgasmic Camel
- Yin Yang

hot tip { Throughout this entire pose, squeeze your lower butt to avoid straining your lower back. Remember to make this a full back bend, not just a severe hinge in your lower back. This pose really intensifies your orgasm while you are either on top or underneath while he's tickling you with his tongue.

MERMAID

This pose deeply stretches and lengthens the abdominal core and the chest. It also tones your butt and glutes while providing a fun posture to perform for your sweetie.

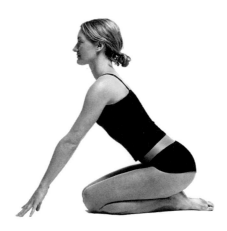

TO DO IT Sitting on your heels with your knees bent, walk your hands forward about three feet.

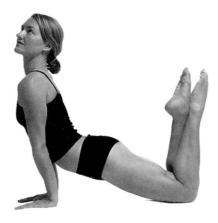

Lean forward with your knees touching, your toes pointed and your back arched. Look up toward the ceiling.

CHAKRAS 3, 5

HOTTIE BODY
- yummy tummy
- yoga butt
- supple spine

IN THE BEDROOM
- Doggie Style
- Orgasmic Camel
- Satisfying Side

hot tip { Strike this flattering pose during your yoga workout or in bed and embrace your sexy inner mermaid. For extra sensual pleasure, try this pose during The Conquest: Simply lower yourself up and down on his penis while bending your knees and squeezing your butt.

LOCUST

This abdominal-strengthening blockbuster also builds serious back strength, combating sway back, sore back, and potbelly. It strongly stimulates the sexual core by squeezing the glutes and the perineum, the "sex strip" located between the anus and the vagina on women and the scrotum on men.

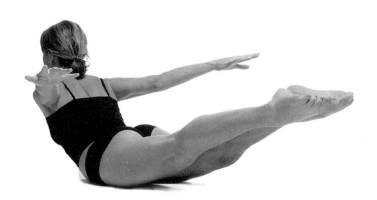

TO DO IT Lie down on your stomach, with your chin resting on the floor and your arms at your sides, palms down. Point your toes, bring your legs together, and squeeze tight to hold your feet together.

Inhale and raise both your torso and your legs off the floor. Raise your arms to your sides like a pair of airplane wings, make your neck long, and gaze a few feet in front of you on the floor. Be sure to straighten your knees, squeeze your legs tight, and lift them as high as you can. Hold for three medium-depth breaths. When finished, rest on the floor with your head turned to one side.

A note of caution: Do not do this pose if you have hypertension, stroke, or heart disease.

VARIATION (INTERMEDIATE) Do as just described, but keep your hands clasped behind your back and your arms lifting as if pulling your torso toward your feet.

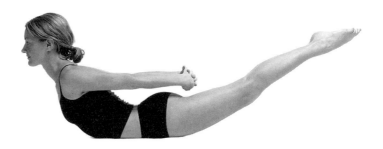

CHAKRAS 2, 3, 4

HOTTIE BODY
· yoga butt
· open chest
· long, lean legs
· sexy shoulders

IN THE BEDROOM
· Bridging the Gap
· Satisfying Side
· Talking in Tongues

hot tip { Squeeze your butt tightly to avoid pinching your back and to increase stimulation of your sexual core. Try having your partner sit on the back of your thighs, close to your butt, and let him gently stretch out your chest and back by holding your shoulders or elbows. Then slowly lean back. You'll feel your sexual core explode with sensation.

FLOOR BOW

This pose strengthens your sexual core and legs while opening your chest and stimulating your endocrine, nervous, circulatory, respiratory, and reproductive systems. It also increases blood flow to your sexual core, heart, spine, and lungs, maintaining healthy ovaries and prostate.

A note of caution: *Do not do this pose if you have hypertension, stroke, or heart disease.*

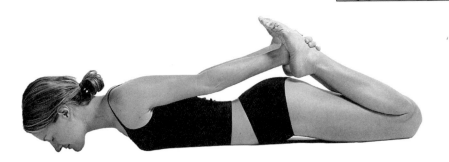

TO DO IT Lie on your stomach with your chin on the floor, arms alongside your body and legs together. Reach back, grasping the inside of your feet with your hands, keeping your feet and toes pointed (see inset). Try to keep your knees close and bring your heels to your butt.

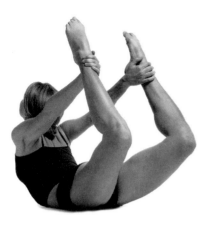

Gently exhale and lift your legs, head, chin, and chest off the floor by pulling on your feet with your hands. The weight of your body should rest on your abdomen. Looking straight ahead, breathe in and out into your sexual core five times. The depth of your back arch depends on how hard you push your legs. To release, exhale and slowly lower your body to the floor, with arms to the side and legs long. Turn your head to one side and rest. Repeat three times.

VARIATION Rock back as you inhale and rock forward as you exhale.

CHAKRAS 2, 3, 4

HOTTIE BODY
- yoga butt
- long, lean legs
- open chest
- sexy shoulders
- yummy tummy

IN THE BEDROOM
- Orgasmic Camel
- Satisfying Side
- Yin Yang

hot tip { Engage your inner thighs by keeping your knees close together. Remember, don't hold your breath! Press your chest forward and contract your abdominal muscles to prevent pinching your lower back. This is an intense "heart opener." Think of your honey and enjoy the flood of love energy in your chest. Remember this pose to improve your Satisfying Side.

PIGEON

This pose stretches the groin, thighs, chest, neck, and shoulders while opening chest to promote better breathing. Men take notice: It is also great for the prostate!

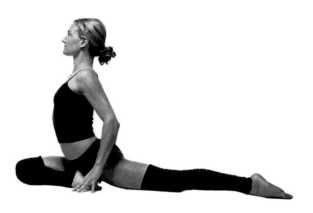

TO DO IT Start in Downward Dog (page 130). Look forward and place your right knee in between your hands. Rest the side of your right leg on the ground and try to decrease the angle of your knee. Lower your left leg straight on the floor behind you, with the top of the foot on floor. Rest your right butt cheek on the floor, and place your fingertips on the floor beneath your shoulders.

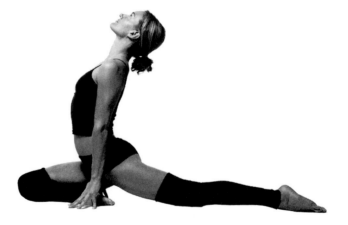

Inhale. Gently pushing through your fingertips, arch your back and look up, feeling the stretch in your chest and hip flexors.

70

Exhale, bend at the waist, and lower your torso onto your right inner thigh. Place your arms on the floor over your head. Breathe out and let yourself feel completely comfortable and relaxed. Breathe in and out into your sexual core five times.

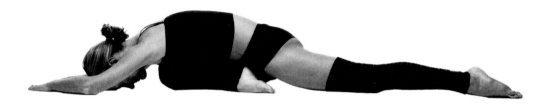

To release, flatten your palms, curl your toes under, and push your torso off the floor into Downward Dog. Repeat on the other side.

VARIATION For a deeper stretch, rise onto the ball of your back foot and flex the leg straight back.

CHAKRAS 1, 4, 6

HOTTIE BODY
· pliable pelvis
· flexible lower back
· open chest
· loose hips

IN THE BEDROOM
· Bundled Package
· Rock Steady
· Splitting Bamboo

hot tip { With some ingenuity, doing this pose while lying on top of your man will bring extra satisfaction to your super-spread hips. Deeply relax and give your hips a chance to release. Yummy!

SLEEPING PIGEON

This is the Pigeon with a twist, literally. This extra move will open your hips further while adding a mid-back twist to dissolve back tension. (If you are pregnant, skip this pose.)

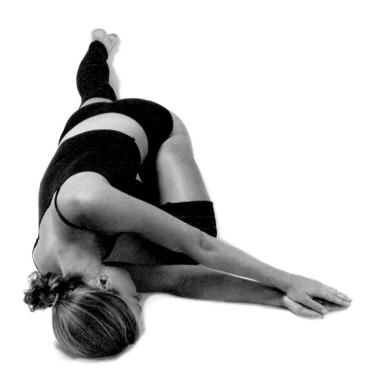

TO DO IT Begin in Pigeon (page 70). Slip your right arm under your left, twisting your back, and place the back of your hand on the floor. Rest your left hand on top of your right and lay your head on the floor.

CHAKRAS 3, 5

HOTTIE BODY
- supple spine
- yoga butt
- pliable pelvis

IN THE BEDROOM
- Backseat Buddies
- Satisfying Side
- Splitting Bamboo

hot tip { The extra twist in the Sleeping Pigeon can help bring deep pleasure for both of you during penetration. Enjoy him inside of you by lying still and simply breathing.

YOGACYCLES *This move tightens your tummy and pelvic floor while bringing flexibility to your mid-back.*

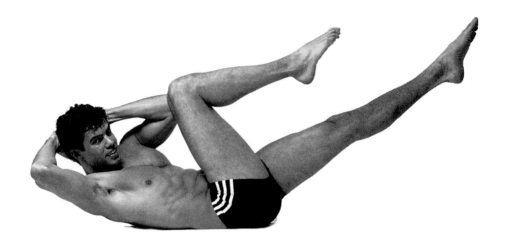

TO DO IT Lie on your back. Clasp your hands lightly behind your neck, being careful not to pull. Bring your right knee in to your chest and your left elbow to your right knee. Raise your left leg about two inches off the floor and point your toes. Switch, bringing your right elbow to your left knee and pushing out your right leg about two inches off of the floor. This is one set. Do fifteen more sets, remembering to breathe deeply in and out of your sexual core.

HOTTIE
BODY
- killer inner thighs
- yummy tummy
- strong obliques

IN THE
BEDROOM
- Satisfying Side
- Surf's Up

hot tip { Keep your back "cemented" to the mat to help isolate the twist in your abdomen, not your shoulders. This pose gets you in great shape—internally—for *all* our sex positions. The internal squeezing required is really a turn-on all by itself. Try it by yourself for instant gratification.

AB SWITCHES
A total body toner, this position creates super-strong abdominal muscles and stimulates sexual core energy.

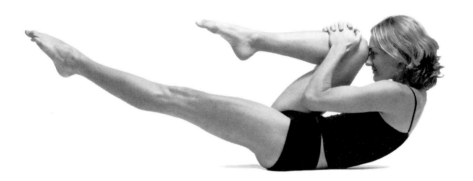

TO DO IT Start by lying on your back. Then bend your right knee toward your chest and interlace your fingers on top of your shin. Next, lift your left leg off the floor, pointing your toes, and lift your back off the floor. Touch your forehead to your knee, squeeze tightly through your core, and hold for four breaths. Repeat on the other side.

CHAKRAS 1, 2, 3, 6

HOTTIE BODY
- yummy tummy
- yoga butt
- gorgeous biceps
- tight triceps

IN THE BEDROOM
- Backseat Buddies
- Satisfying Side

hot tip { This pose puts you in great shape, internally, for *all* of the bedroom positions. The internal squeezing required is really a turn-on all by itself. Try it!

BALLET BELLY
This pose tightens your tummy and pelvic floor while sculpting the inner thighs. Think long, sleek, and sexy like a ballerina.

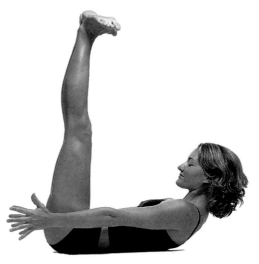

TO DO IT

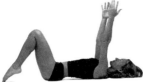

Lie flat on your back. Inhale, bend your knees, and raise your arms above you toward the ceiling. Keep your pelvis tilted forward, allowing for space under your lower back.

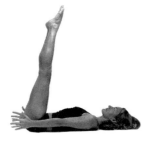

Exhale and raise your legs straight up toward the ceiling with your toes pointed. Lower your hands to the sides of your legs. Now tilt your pelvis backward so that your back is nice and flat on the floor.

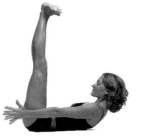

Inhale and lift your shoulder blades from the floor, flex your feet, and rotate your legs outward like a ballet dancer.

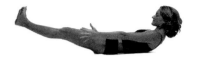

Exhale and slowly lower your legs, using your abs, until they almost touch (but don't) the floor. Hold here for two full breaths while gazing at your feet. After about five seconds, release and relax completely on your back for two breaths. Repeat eight times.

CHAKRAS 1, 2, 5

HOTTIE BODY
- killer inner thighs
- yoga butt
- yummy tummy

IN THE BEDROOM
- Rock Steady

hot tip {
Really engage your inner thighs and keep your lower back firmly on the ground. After you practice these tummy-toners daily, you'll be delighted to show off your midriff.

KARATE BODY

A traditional movement practiced in martial arts training, this abdominal exercise works to both strengthen and center your entire body, particularly your core.

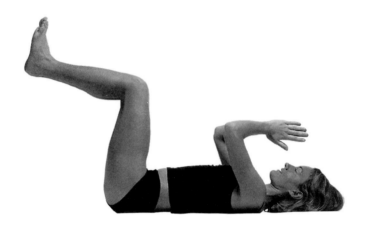

TO DO IT Lie on your back with both knees bent and palms together on the center of your breastbone. Keep your feet flexed with your ankles touching.

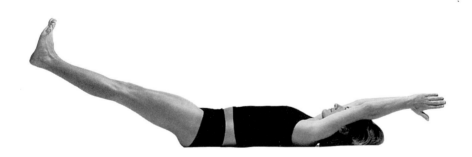

Inhale and, at the same time, raise both arms above your head and both legs straight out in front of you. Keep your arms and legs lifted off the floor about six inches. Pause, then exhale and return to the starting position with your arms and legs bent. Repeat sixteen times.

CHAKRAS 2, 5

HOTTIE BODY
- yoga butt
- yummy tummy
- killer inner thighs

IN THE BEDROOM
- Bathing Beauties
- Surf's Up
- Talking in Tongues
- Wild Child

hot tip { For best results, keep your ankles touching and your legs completely straight when you extend them forward. Also, use your core strength, not your leg muscles, to raise and lower your legs. You'll find this position realigns your heart and sexual energies, making you a better lover—and partner.

CHA CHA CHA *This sexy, flexy Latin dance move beautifies the inner thighs, shapes the waist, and defines the obliques.*

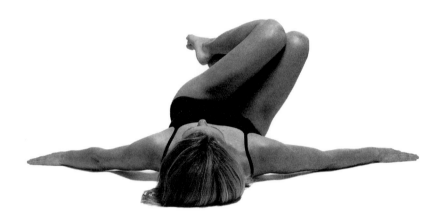

TO DO IT Lie on your back, as if your back is cemented on the floor. Keep your arms at a 45-degree angle by your sides, with your palms facing down. Bend your knees to your chest and squeeze them tightly together.

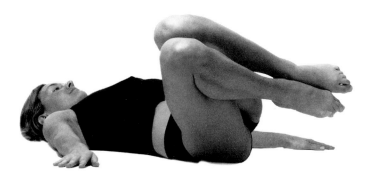

Drop both legs to the right as if to skim the ground with your right knee. Pull both legs up, through center, and over to other side in a figure-eight form. Repeat on the left side. Finish with a quick figure-eight left, right, left. Slow–Slow, Quick–Quick–Quick. CHA CHA CHA CHA CHA!

HOTTIE BODY
- whittled waistline
- strong obliques
- yummy tummy
- killer inner thighs

IN THE BEDROOM
- Bathing Beauties
- Bundled Package
- Doggie Style
- Wild Child

hot tip { Remember to keep your inner knees touching at all times so that you can develop those gorgeous oblique muscles. This nontraditional pose brings out your inner diva and gets your hips ready to gyrate.

PELVIC SQUEEZES
These tiny squeezes seriously hit the spot! This move, which isolates and tightens the sexual core, can be an effective form of foreplay, as you contract many of the same muscles involved in orgasm. Practice this one whenever you can.

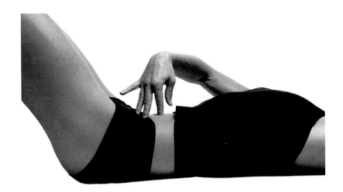

TO DO IT While lying on your back, touch your feet and knees together and place your arms above your head, resting on the floor. Isolate the muscles beneath your belly button and in the pelvic girdle—the sexual core muscles—and tuck your pelvis under slightly to get your back flat on the ground.

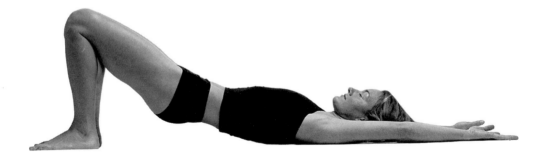

Now that your back is flat, lift your tailbone and sacrum (the large triangular bone at the base of your spine and upper part of your pelvis) up off the floor slightly, squeezing your inner thighs, then lower. Completely relax all the muscles. Inhale and lift up again, exhale and lower. Repeat sixteen times. Remember to breathe in and out of your sexual core as you raise and lower your pelvis.

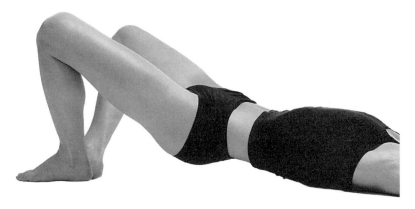

For your second set of sixteen, repeat the same basic movement but open your knees wide while keeping your feet together. For your third set of sixteen, repeat with your knees touching and your feet wide.

CHAKRAS 1, 2

HOTTIE BODY
· yoga butt
· long, lean legs

IN THE BEDROOM
· Bridging the Gap
· The Conquest
· Wild Child
· Yin Yang

hot tip { This is a micromovement. Do not exaggerate it. Gaining awareness and control over these subtle yet vital muscles will help you achieve greater sexual energy and control.

BUMP BUMP BUMP
This steamy and stimulating move brings both energy and blood flow to your sexual core and sacrum, and develops your pelvic flexibility.

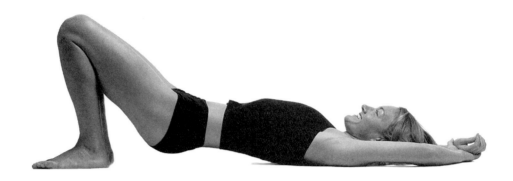

TO DO IT Begin by lying on your back, with your feet flat on the floor and hips lifted. Keep your buttocks and belly firm.

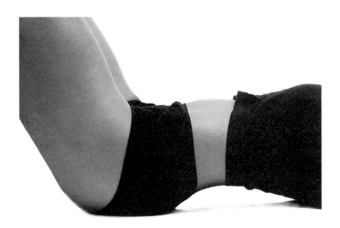

Drop your lower back slightly, exaggerating the curve there. Very gently bump your sacrum to the floor three times quickly. Then raise your hips off the floor and hold for three seconds. Repeat sixteen times while keeping your breath regular and calm.

CHAKRAS 1, 2

HOTTIE BODY
- yoga butt
- yummy tummy
- killer inner thighs

IN THE BEDROOM
- Bridging the Gap
- The Conquest
- Rock Steady

hot tip { This is a killer move to try with your partner during sex. A warning: It arouses both of you quickly, so use it only when you're both ready.

BELLY ROLL
What a fabulous move! It establishes muscle control throughout your back and abdomen, allowing for pelvic flexibility; it also soothes tight groins. Usually done before and after a Half Bridge or Bridge as a back release in yoga, it can also be incorporated into the sex position Surf's Up.

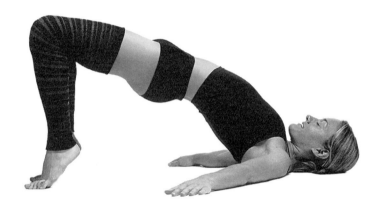

TO DO IT Lie on your back with your knees bent, feet separated a few inches and your arms by your sides. Lift your pelvis high off the floor beginning at the sacrum and moving up the spine toward your shoulder blades.

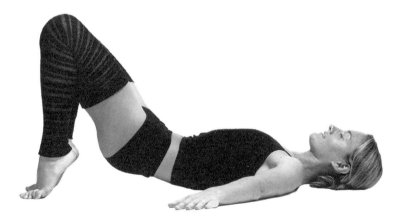

Pause, then reverse the roll through your spine, beginning at the top of your back and moving toward the sacrum. Feel each vertebra touch the floor one at a time, gently controlling the speed and saving your tailbone for last.

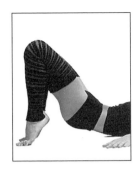

Remember to elongate your back by pushing your tailbone toward your knees as you roll your spine down the floor.

CHAKRAS 1, 2, 3, 4

HOTTIE BODY
- yoga butt
- yummy tummy
- killer inner thighs

IN THE BEDROOM
- Bridging the Gap
- Bundled Package
- The Conquest
- Orgasmic Camel
- Rearview

hot tip { As mentioned, try to roll down slowly, one vertebra at a time. You've got to try this one when your man is on top in The Conquest! Don't be surprised if he begs for you to move faster, but we suggest giving it to him nice and slow. You don't want him coming too soon.

HALF BRIDGE

This pose builds a strong sexual core and lower body by lengthening and strengthening your abdomen, pelvis, and chest. It also energizes your body by stimulating your endocrine and nervous systems.

A note of caution: *This pose is not recommended for anyone who is hypertensive, on hypertension medication, or suffers from a heart condition.*

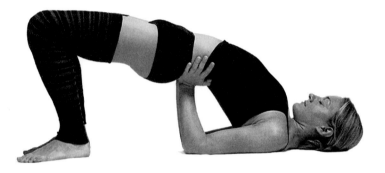

TO DO IT

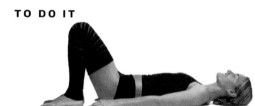

Lie flat on your back. Bend both knees and place your feet close to your butt, flat on the floor and hip width apart. Slide your arms alongside your body with your palms facing down, fingertips close to your heels.

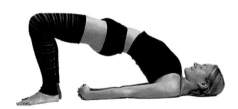

Lift your pelvis off the ground, with your hips toward the ceiling, and tuck your chin to your chest. Walk your shoulder blades together underneath your back and clasp your fingers beneath the lower back. Breathe in and out of your sexual core five times.

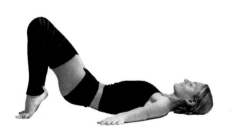

To release, rise onto the balls of your feet, unclasp your hands, roll your shoulders out, and very slowly lower your back to the ground. Use your abdominal strength to press your spine, one vertebra at a time, back to the floor.

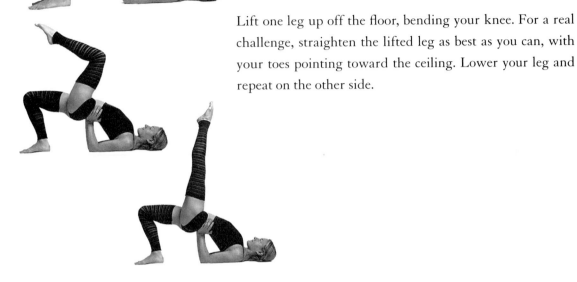

VARIATIONS (INTERMEDIATE) Instead of interlacing the fingers under your back, place your hands under the small of your back and let the weight of your pelvis rest on your hands.

Lift one leg up off the floor, bending your knee. For a real challenge, straighten the lifted leg as best as you can, with your toes pointing toward the ceiling. Lower your leg and repeat on the other side.

CHAKRAS 2, 3, 4, 5, 7

HOTTIE BODY
- flexible lower back
- yummy tummy
- yoga butt
- killer inner thighs

IN THE BEDROOM
- Bridging the Gap
- Orgasmic Camel
- Rearview

hot tip { When preparing to move into the Bridge, squeeze your knees close together, but not touching, as the knees tend to splay sideways in the pose—this will help you to better target your sexual core. Let your knees relax out to the sides a bit, making room for your partner to scoot in between.

BRIDGE
This pose may take some time to build up to, but it is so worth it! It encourages the natural flow of sexual energy to move up the center of the torso and to the top of your head. The pose also tones the rear, abdomen, legs, and arms.

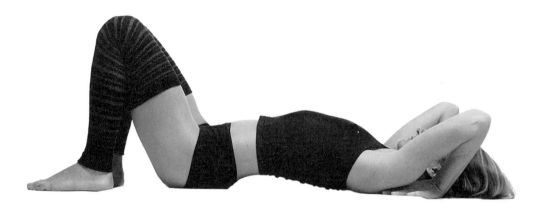

TO DO IT Lie flat on your back. Bend both knees and place your feet close to your butt, flat on the floor and hip width apart. Place your palms on the floor underneath your shoulders.

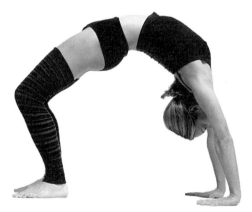

Push your shoulders into the ground and straighten your arms. At the same time, exhale and lift your pelvis off the floor into a full back bend. (A full back bend arches the whole back, not just the lower back.) Imagine a strap tied around your mid-back pulling you off the floor, making the highest point of the bend just above your belly button. Try to point the crown of your head toward your heels with your face looking at the floor. Straighten your arms and keep your fingers spread wide, without letting your elbows fly out sideways. Breathe in deeply and establish a connection between your chest and sexual core. To release, tuck your chin to your chest and gently lower your back to the floor slowly, using the Belly Roll.

CHAKRAS 2, 3, 4, 5, 7

HOTTIE BODY
- flexible lower back
- yummy tummy
- yoga butt
- killer inner thighs

IN THE BEDROOM
- Bridging the Gap
- Orgasmic Camel
- Rearview

hot tip {
Remember to breathe! Holding your breath only makes this pose more difficult. Try to arch your whole back, as this lessens the weight-bearing load on your arms. If you dare, try this pose while your partner stands above you. Trust us, he'll get so excited he may even start pleasuring you. But don't do this on the bed; you'll need a harder surface for your arms and wrists to remain strong.

SEATED FORWARD BEND
This move tones your leg muscles while stretching your hamstrings and lower back for ultimate flexibility.

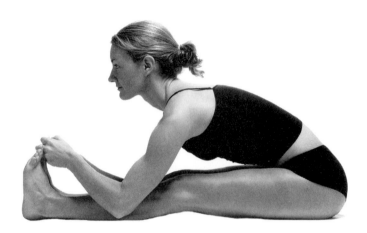

TO DO IT Seated on the floor, flex your feet, keep your back straight, raise your arms in the air, and bend forward with your chin lifted. Look forward, and interlace your fingers around your big toes. Make sure to keep flexing your feet. Pull your body forward and hold for five deep breaths.

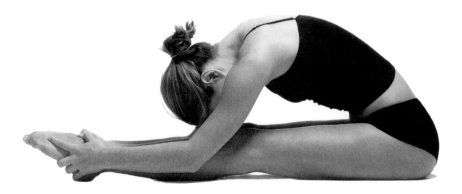

Point your feet and drop your head forward, relaxing the back of your neck. Feel the delicious stretch in the upper back and neck.

CHAKRAS 1, 2, 5

HOTTIE BODY
- long, lean legs
- tight triceps
- gorgeous biceps
- yummy tummy
- flexible lower back

IN THE BEDROOM
- Backward-Forward Bend
- Bathing Beauties
- Rearview
- Splitting Bamboo

hot tip {

Keep your legs taut with your knees pressed into the floor, thigh muscles flexed and legs squeezing together. Then keep your legs "active" by flexing your thigh muscles and straightening your knees. This can be a fun one to try while sitting atop of your very erect partner facing his feet. Let him take hold of your hips and rock you back and forth.

IN THE SADDLE
This pose opens your hips and stretches your legs, back, and shoulders. It also regulates the adrenal glands and stimulates Ming Men—*an acupressure point named "the gate of life," where sexual energy is stored.*

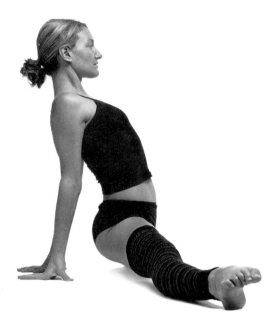

TO DO IT

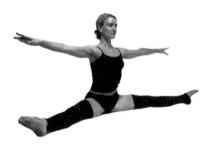

Start from a seated position, legs outstretched in front of you. Open your legs as wide as you can and point your feet out.

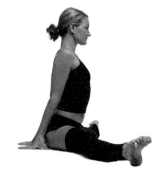

Place your hands behind your butt, and push up onto your fingers, lengthening and straightening your entire back. Pull your shoulders back and keep them low. Hold this position and feel a deep opening in your inner thighs and hips. Make sure your back is always straight. Do not go to the next stage until you can move your hands to the inside of your thighs without your back collapsing.

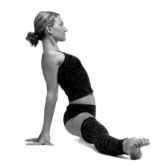

Place your hands behind your butt and, while lifting up, press your hips forward, getting as much inner thigh stretch as possible. Keep your back flat.

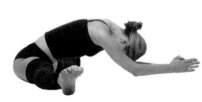

Walk your hands forward between your legs, then walk your elbows forward, moving your belly as low to the floor as you can. Use your forearms to pull you forward. Breathe in and out into your sexual core five times. To release, walk your arms back in and bring your legs together. Shake your legs out in front of you.

CHAKRAS 3, 5

HOTTIE BODY
• sexy shoulders
• long, lean legs
• pliable pelvis

IN THE BEDROOM
• Erotic Froggie
• Oops, I Dropped the Soap!
• Rock Steady
• Talking in Tongues

hot tip { Press the back of your knees into the floor and keep your legs engaged and taut, as if you were standing. This will further stimulate Ming Men and help release sexual energy.

SIDESADDLE

A deep stretch, this pose really tones the inner thighs while opening the hips in a big way.

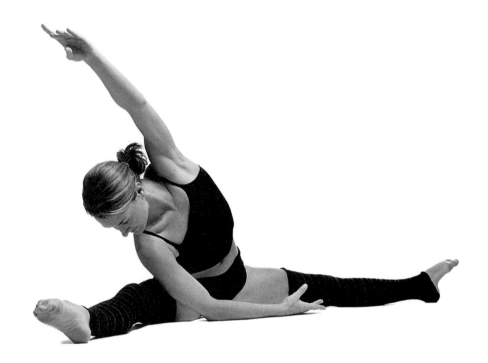

TO DO IT Start in In the Saddle (page 96). Keeping your butt on the floor, reach your left arm up and over your head toward your right leg, with your right arm reaching on the floor toward your left leg. Keep your chest open and gaze at your feet. Hold for five breaths. Repeat on the other side.

CHAKRAS 1, 2, 3

HOTTIE · loose hips
BODY · killer inner thighs

· whittled waistline

· yummy tummy

· open chest

IN THE · Rock Steady
BEDROOM · Satisfying Side

hot tip { With this much flexibility in your hips, imagine all the fun positions in bed you can try.

TABLETOP

This pose is another great one for firming the butt and abs; it also strengths your sexual core and opens your chest. In addition, it releases blocked energy in the throat chakra (number five), allowing for expressive communication.

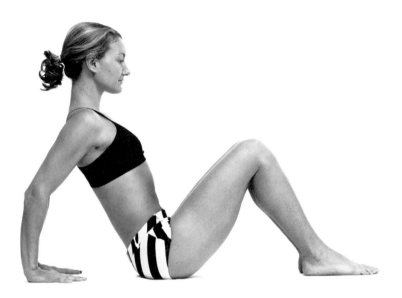

TO DO IT Sit on the floor with your feet hip width apart, knees bent and your hands behind you, fingertips facing your rear. Lift your hips off the floor and bring your thighs in line with your abs and torso.

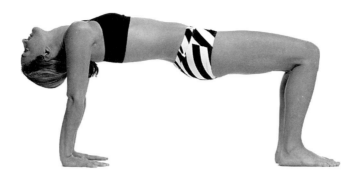

Keep your knees positioned directly above your ankles and squeeze your inner thighs to prevent your knees from spreading open. Release your head backward and relax your throat.

CHAKRAS 1, 2, 5

HOTTIE BODY
· yummy tummy
· yoga butt
· sexy arms

IN THE BEDROOM
· The Conquest
· Mermaid
· Surf's Up
· Wild Child

hot tip { Make your body flat like a tabletop by lifting your tailbone and chest up to really open up your fifth chakra. Expressive communication with your partner makes for better lovemaking; you can tell him exactly what you want—and don't.

FLASHDANCE

The yoga version of the hot pose made famous by Jennifer Beals in the movie Flashdance *is sure to rev up your yoga workout—and your sex life. This pose tones your abs, inner thighs, and calves while opening your chest and throat. It also releases tension in the chest, making room for more love.*

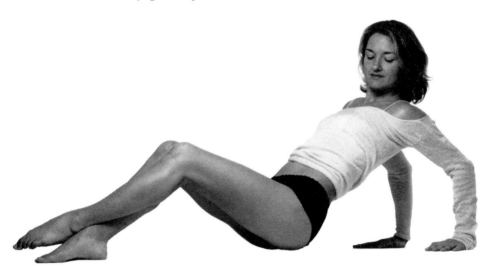

TO DO IT Begin seated on the floor, with both legs stretched out in front of you and your hands under your shoulders with fingertips facing your rear. Cross your left ankle over your right one and shift your weight onto the right leg. Lift your hips up, make your tummy flat, and keep your legs straight.

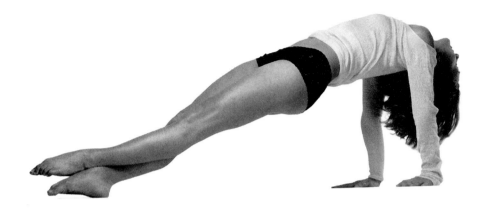

Open your chest toward the ceiling and release your head back, relaxing the front of your throat. Hold here for two breaths. Then bend your knees, lower your hips halfway back to the starting position, and breathe two breaths into your sexual core.

CHAKRAS 2, 3, 4, 5

HOTTIE BODY
- killer inner thighs
- yummy tummy
- yoga butt
- tight triceps

IN THE BEDROOM
- Bridging the Gap
- The Conquest
- Splitting Bamboo

hot tip { Squeeze your butt and your inner thighs, and keep your core strong. Not only is this a sexy pose to watch, but it makes for an interesting change in the sack. Be on top, face the ceiling, and lower yourself up and down on top of your ready, willing, and able partner.

KILLER HIP OPENER
This "killer" pose stretches the hips, glutes, and hamstrings while sending a rush of blood to your muscles in this area. Practicing this pose consistently can help to eliminate years of blocked energy in the pelvis. After you unblock this energy, you can expect increased sexual arousal, heightened genital sensitivity, and even an emotional release.

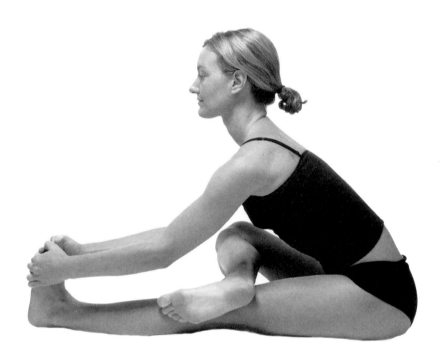

TO DO IT Sit on the floor with your legs together extended out in front of you. Cross your right leg on top of your left thigh, with your right ankle outside of your lower left knee. Flex both feet, exhale, and bend forward from the waist toward your bent leg. Breathe in and out of your sexual core five times. Release and repeat on the other side.

CHAKRAS 1, 2, 3

HOTTIE
BODY
· loose hips
· pliable pelvis
· long, lean legs

IN THE
BEDROOM
· Backseat Buddies
· Erotic Froggie
· Rock Steady
· Splitting Bamboo

hot tip { This is an intense hip opener. Go to your limit and breathe deeply into any tight areas while pulling your torso toward your foot. Feel free to sway your body from side to side while working out tight spots. Make sure both ankles are flexed. You'll appreciate this release in your hips later, believe us!

DIAMOND
This pose provides a great stretch to the front of your thighs and increases flexibility in your knees, hips, and spine.

TO DO IT

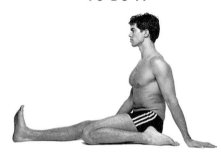

From a seated position with your legs straight out in front of you, bend your left knee so that your heel is as close to your thigh as possible and the top of your foot is flat on the floor. Keep your right leg extended and flexed.

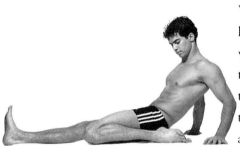

With your knees close together, slowly and carefully walk your hands behind you, lowering your back toward the floor. Start with your elbows one at a time, then, if you can, lower your entire back to the floor. Go only as far as you feel comfortable, then hold and breathe in and out five times. To release, hold on to your ankles or feet and press into your elbows, using your arms to lift your head and torso back up and off the floor. When coming out of this posture, be mindful of your knees: Go slowly, and if you need to, massage your knees to refresh the blood flow to the area. Repeat on the other side.

VARIATION (INTERMEDIATE)

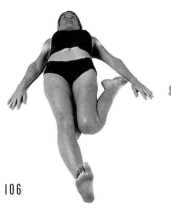

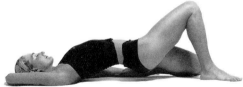

Lie on your back as before but now bend your left leg and place the sole of your foot on the floor. Then lift your butt cheek off the floor by pressing into your standing leg. Twist your pelvis inward to get the best stretch in your hip and top of your thigh.

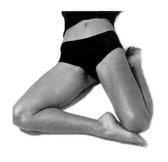

Push the bent knee that is resting on the floor down to feel a deeper stretch in your quad and your pelvis. Then try pushing the knee to the inside of your body and to the outside. Hold for a few breaths in each position, working out any kinks or tight spots in your sexual core and the surrounding muscles.

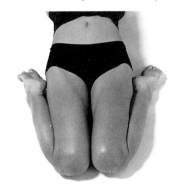

FULL DIAMOND

Standing on your knees, lower your butt down to your heels and then spread your heels so your butt touches the floor. Keeping your knees close together, slowly and carefully walk your hands behind you, lowering your back toward the floor. Lower one elbow at a time to the floor; then, if you can, lower your back to the floor. Your hips should be parallel to the floor. Breathe in and out of your sexual core five times. To release, hold on to your ankles or feet and press into your elbows, using your arms to lift your head and torso off the floor. Walk your hands back to your hips, and return to the starting position.

CHAKRAS 2, 3

HOTTIE BODY	**IN THE BEDROOM**
· pliable pelvis	· Erotic Froggie
· yoga butt	· Wild Child
· flexible knees	

hot tip {

Keep your abs and glutes tight while positioning your tailbone toward your knees. While in this pose, if your butt doesn't reach the floor, use a yoga block or a blanket to prop it up. Do *not* lean back. Feel free to massage your knees and thighs. The gentle stretching of the knees and hips afforded by this pose will make the good old missionary position—or The Conquest—a lot more comfortable.

BUTTERFLY

A terrific anxiety and fatigue fighter, this move lengthens the spine and stimulates the reproductive, circulatory, nervous, and respiratory systems. It also increases blood flow to your legs and pelvis and keeps the kidneys and bladder healthy.

TO DO IT

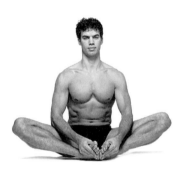

Starting from a seated position, bring the soles of your feet together with your knees bent out to the sides like a butterfly. Clasp your fingers around your feet. Inhale and stretch the top of your head toward the ceiling with your chin down toward your chest. Drop your shoulders down and back. Press your chest out toward the wall in front of you while keeping your back flat. Breathe in and out of your sexual core five times.

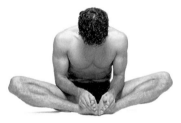

For a deeper stretch, round your back, squeezing in your abs and using your arms to help pull your upper body towards your toes. At the same time, place your elbows on your inner thighs and press them down to the floor while bringing your forehead toward your toes, relaxing your head and neck.

VARIATION

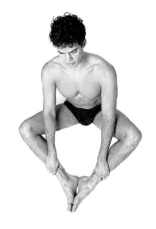

Scoot your feet farther out in front of you, so your legs make a diamond shape. Keep the soles of your feet touching.

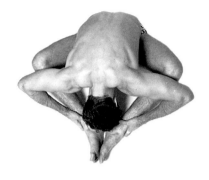

Bend at the waist, bringing your chin toward the floor.

CHAKRAS 1, 2, 6, 7

HOTTIE BODY
· pliable pelvis and hamstrings
· flexible lower back

IN THE BEDROOM
· Bathing Beauties
· Bridging the Gap
· Erotic Froggie
· Talking in Tongues

hot tip { Spread the soles of your feet open by pushing thumbs into the balls of the feet under the big toes. Inch by inch, walk your thumbs from your arches up the inside of the leg all the way to your groin. This encourages the flow of yin energy to your kidneys, where your sexual energy is stored.

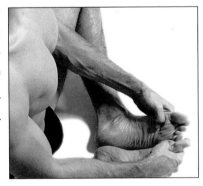

SEXY SPINAL TWIST

This move feels great anytime and anywhere. It can even be done while seated in your chair. You'll see that later on, in the section titled "Sexy Secretary Poses." This pose stretches the obliques and abdomen while getting the kinks out of your shoulders and back.

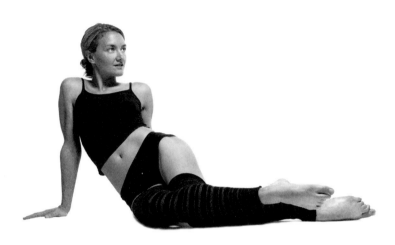

TO DO IT

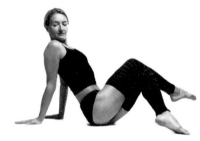

Sit with your knees bent and feet on the floor. Walk your hands behind you a foot or so, and cross your right knee over your left.

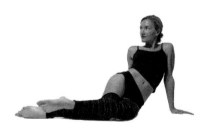

Inhale, then exhale, twist, and lower your knees toward the left side and gently twist, looking over your shoulder. (This is a great move when a lover is watching.)

110

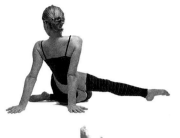

Extend your top leg straight and look back over your shoulder. Inhale, move back to the center, and then exhale and drop to the other side, looking over your opposite shoulder. Repeat eight times, then, when centered, uncross your legs.

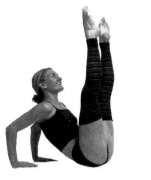

Point both feet toward the ceiling, squeeze your tummy and sexual core, and hold for two breaths. Return to the starting position and repeat on the opposite side.

CHAKRAS 2, 3, 4

HOTTIE BODY
- whittled waist
- yoga butt
- sexy shoulders

IN THE BEDROOM
- Backseat Buddies
- Rearview
- Satisfying Side

hot tip { **Use your shoulders to facilitate a deeper twist in your torso. If you try this twist during Rearview, be careful not to rest your weight on your man's midsection.**

SEATED FOREHEAD TO KNEE

This amazing pose both strengthens the abs and stretches the heck out of your hamstrings and glute muscles.

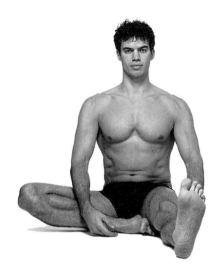

TO DO IT In a sitting position, open your left leg to the side 45 degrees and bend your right knee, bringing the sole of your right foot to your left inner thigh.

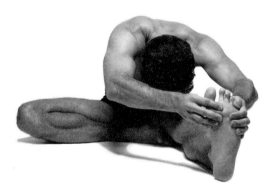

Reach out and forward (using a towel wrapped around your foot if you can't reach your toes) and interlace your hands under your left foot. Pull yourself down and tuck your forehead to your right kneecap (or in the direction of your knee). Contract your upper abdominal muscles for control, and try to keep your shoulders level.

CHAKRAS 1, 2, 3

HOTTIE
BODY
- yoga butt
- yummy tummy
- long, lean legs
- sexy shoulders and arms

———————————

IN THE
BEDROOM
- Backward-Forward Bend
- Bundled Package
- Oops, I Dropped the Soap!
- Splitting Bamboo
- Talking in Tongues

hot tip { Keeping your shoulders even requires that you involve your abdominal muscles. Don't just bend forward and let your stomach spill over; lift up your abdomen and then twist slightly. Your partner will surely appreciate those twisty moves, which help to add deeper stimulation.

HALF BACK BEND

Usually following the Seated Fore-head to Knee pose, this partial back bend feels amazing and is an easy way to stretch out the front of your torso and hip flexors. It's also a safer stretch for those who can't do a full back bend.

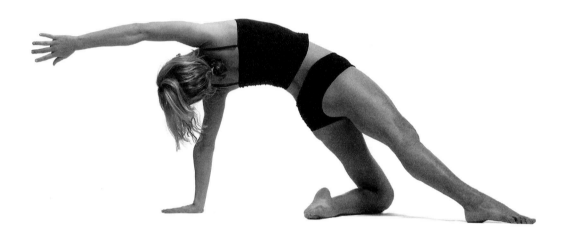

TO DO IT Seated with your left knee bent and right leg extended, lift your butt off the floor and reach your right arm over your head and behind you. Balance on your left hand and knee. Stretch out the front of your torso while arching your back for five breaths. Then lower back down and repeat on the other side.

CHAKRAS 2, 3, 4, 5

HOTTIE BODY
- flexible lower back
- loose hips
- yummy tummy
- sexy shoulders and arms

IN THE BEDROOM
- Orgasmic Camel
- Talking in Tongues

hot tip { Trust us when we say this pose can be a useful stretch while performing Talking in Tongues.

ALMOST LOTUS

This is a fantastic stretch for tight hips and glutes. It can free up blocked energy in the pelvis by stimulating your second chakra and the perineum. Don't worry, you don't have to be a pretzel to enjoy all the benefits of this pose.

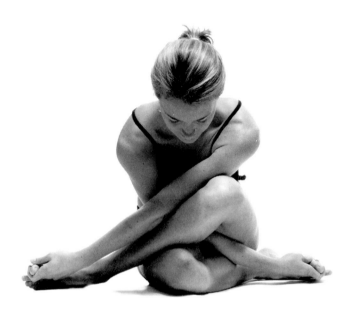

TO DO IT Begin by sitting on the floor. Point your right knee straight ahead, cross your left leg over your right, and reach your right hand under your left leg to your right foot. With your left hand, hold on to your left toe and squeeze all your toes on each foot. Your knees do not need to be perfectly one on top of the other. Make your back straight and then bend at the waist, looking straight ahead. When you've reached as far as you can comfortably go, release your head forward, relaxing the back of your neck.

CHAKRAS 1, 2, 3, 4, 5

HOTTIE BODY
- loose hips
- sexy back
- relaxed neck

IN THE BEDROOM
- Backseat Buddies
- Bundled Package

hot tip {

Keep both butt cheeks on the floor. The tendency to favor one side over the other will prevent you from achieving a really amazing hip stretch. Your natural curves and/or athletic legs will probably keep your knees from touching—and that's okay. Just make sure to keep both butt cheeks on the floor for an amazing hip stretch. This is another great pose for helping you get down in cramped spaces.

BOAT

This bold move floods your pelvis with energy and blood. It stimulates the perineum and builds power and strength where it matters most—in the sexual core. Can you think of a better warm-up for sex?

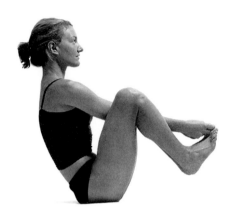

TO DO IT Sit on your butt with your knees bent. Using the index and middle finger of each hand, hold each of your big toes.

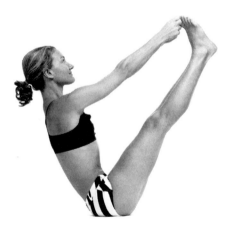

Roll back onto your sit bones (the pelvic bones in your bottom that get sore after sitting at length on a hard chair) while you straighten your legs forward and up diagonally. Your arms, back, and legs should be straight with feet flexed, chin down to elongate your upper back. Balance and hold for five breaths.

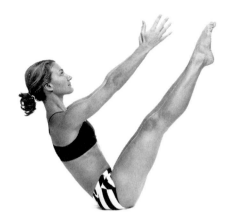

VARIATION If you cannot touch your toes, then simply reach your hands up and point them toward your feet. Keep squeezing in your sexual core and lifting your perineum.

CHAKRAS 1, 2, 3, 4

HOTTIE BODY
· yummy tummy
· long, lean legs
· perfect posture
· open chest

IN THE BEDROOM
· Backseat Buddies
· Bathing Beauties
· Rock Steady

hot tip { Slightly pressing your toes into your fingers creates an isometric stretch so that it's easier to get your legs straighter. We love the Boat for its extra simulation and tingling in your genitals and perineum. Practice really does make perfect for this sexy pose.

WIND-RELIEVING
This pose does just what it says—so do it when your partner isn't around! The move massages your digestive system, releasing any gas that's stored up in your intestines, and also stretches the lower back and opens the hip sockets.

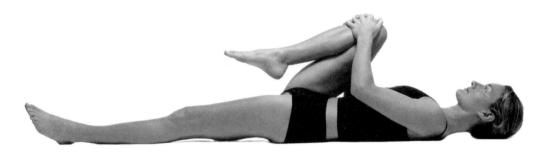

TO DO IT Lie on your back with your legs straight and arms by your sides. Bend your right knee to your chest, interlacing your fingers below your kneecap, and pull your knee toward your right shoulder. Hold the position and take five deep breaths, expanding your lower back and abdomen. Keep both legs totally relaxed and both shoulders on the floor. Relax everything except your arms. This will encourage the wind to pass. Release and repeat on the other side.

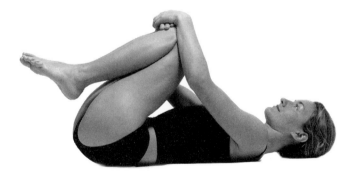

Bring both knees to your chest and wrap your arms around both legs in a hug. Hold, breathe, and release any hip and pelvic tension. Breathe into and out of your sexual core five times.

CHAKRAS 1, 2, 3

HOTTIE BODY
- sexy arms
- yummy tummy
- loose hips

IN THE BEDROOM
- Bathing Beauties
- Bundled Package
- Splitting Bamboo
- Talking in Tongues

hot tip { Touch both shoulders to the floor. Always keep your legs and hips relaxed, letting your arms do the work. Slightly tuck your chin to chest to elongate your neck and eliminate any stored-up gas so that you are more comfortable later, when it really matters.

OF GREAT BENEFIT

This move feels amazing no matter how many times you've done it. It stretches the hips, thighs, hamstrings, groin, and calves while clearing your mind and helping to relieve menstrual discomfort.

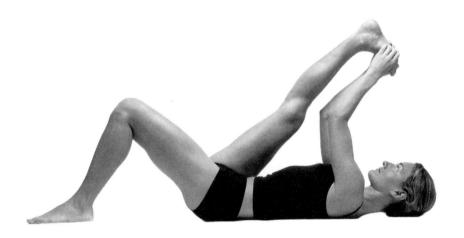

TO DO IT Lie on your back, bend your left knee, and place the sole of your foot on the floor. Extend your right leg up to the ceiling, flexing your foot. Hold underneath the bottom of your foot (use a towel or strap if you can't reach your foot comfortably). Keep your leg perfectly straight, and gently pull the leg in the direction of your forehead, keeping your back on the floor.

CHAKRAS 1, 2, 3

HOTTIE BODY
- long, lean legs
- flexible lower back
- loose hips
- pliable pelvis

IN THE BEDROOM
- Backward-Forward Bend
- Bundled Package
- Double Triangle
- Splitting Bamboo

hot tip { How far your leg reaches toward your forehead is not as important as is the feeling of release in the back of your leg and lower back. That's what really counts. Your leg over your lover's shoulder (Splitting Bamboo) will ensure deep satisfaction to both of you.

EASY SPINAL TWIST

Used chiefly as a gentle stretch to twist your whole back, this is a great way to cool down after moving through some tough positions (even sexual ones!).

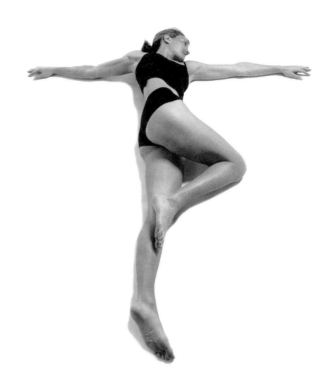

TO DO IT Lie on your back and bring your arms up to shoulder height, palms facing down. Bend your right knee, while keeping your left leg straight, and roll over onto your left side. Turn your head in the same direction, with your chin near your left shoulder. Breathe deeply into your lower back five times. (This will help release pelvic tension.) Repeat on the other side.

CHAKRAS 2, 3, 4, 5

HOTTIE BODY
- supple spine
- sexy lower back
- whittled waist
- relaxed neck
- loose hips

IN THE BEDROOM
- Double Triangle
- Mermaid
- Satisfying Side

hot tip { Be calm, and don't force or strain your back when you do this pose. Stretching out your hips, back, and rear will give your bedroom buddy a great view!

REAR RELEASE
This is a great butt stretch that lengthens your glutes and opens your hips.

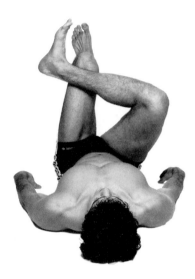

TO DO IT Lie on your back, tucking your pelvis under so that you can feel the small of your back making contact with the floor. Bend your right knee and cross the ankle above the left kneecap.

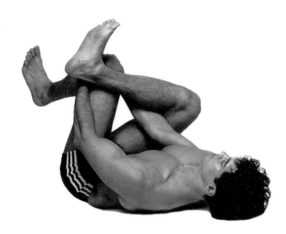

Interlace your fingers on top of your shin bone. Gently pull your left knee toward your chest and try to keep the right shin parallel to the floor. Breathe in and out five times. Uncross your hands and legs and then repeat on the other side.

CHAKRAS 1, 2

HOTTIE BODY
· yoga butt

_____

IN THE BEDROOM
· Bundled Package
· Double Triangle
· Oops, I Dropped the Soap!

hot tip ⎰ Try to keep your shoulders touching the floor and your hips relaxed. Make sure your back is flat on the floor and that your chin is slightly tucked toward your chest. This will give you an unbelievable rear stretch for deep stimulation.

AT PEACE

This pose calms the mind and relieves stress and depression. It also lowers blood pressure and is great for headaches and fatigue. At Peace is the last pose in every yoga routine, and it's meant to settle the deep changes inside your body after a yoga workout, facilitating the free flow of energy and circulation.

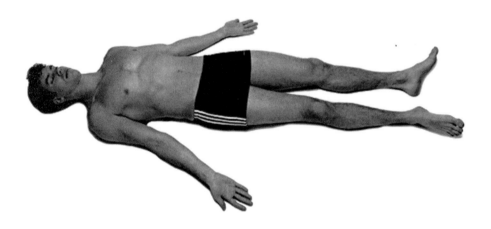

TO DO IT Lie flat on your back, legs straight, with your feet loose and relaxed. Your palms should be facing up with your arms slightly away from your body. Tuck your shoulders down and in, away from your neck. Keep your eyes closed, and sink into the floor. Scan your body for any tension, and breathe deeply in and out five times, then relax your breathing to normal and calm. Relax your eyes; your jaw, mouth, and tongue; and let your forehead be smooth and free of wrinkles. Your arms and legs should feel heavy and warm. Once you find your position, resist the urge to move or fidget, even if you have an itch. Let it pass, and watch how thoughts and emotions come and go. Don't dwell on any one in particular. Let your mind and body be free.

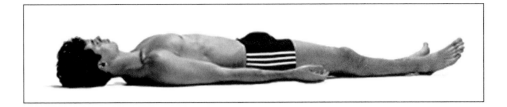

If you have time, stay in this position until you feel all the tension in your face completely release. When people say someone has a "yoga glow," it's often because the person has mastered this position.

CHAKRAS All chakras, large and small!

HOTTIE BODY
- wrinkle remover
- sexy shoulders and arms
- open chest
- loose hips
- supple spine

IN THE BEDROOM
- The Conquest
- Talking in Tongues
- Yin Yang

hot tip { The hardest part of this pose is keeping your body and mind still without fidgeting. But work at it—it's an excellent frame of mind to adopt while receiving oral sex.

STANDING POSES

Standing poses build balance, strength, and flexibility. As you balance, try focusing on the sexual energy in your core. Then feel that energy flow throughout your entire body. Once you've mastered a few of the more challenging standing poses, such as Half Moon (page 158) and Standing Beau (page 170), you may want to try sex while standing on your feet rather than lying on your back. Believe it or not, most women have never tried sex while standing! It's a great alternative and will definitely add variety to your bedroom fun. (You can try standing sex in every room of your house!)

DOWNWARD DOG

This pose is one of the most important basic yoga building blocks. It stretches your back, Achilles' heels, and the backs of your legs while opening your chest and building upper body strength. It also stimulates your sexual core, brain, and nervous system, and improves your memory, concentration, and sexual energy, all the while increasing blood flow to your head and heart.

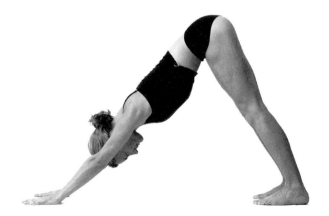

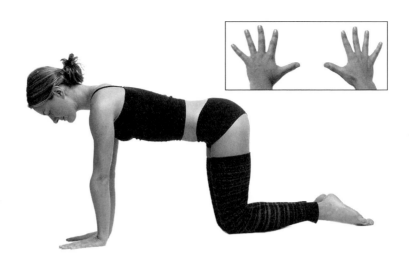

TO DO IT Begin in On All Fours (page 50). Keep your fingers wide apart with your middle finger facing forward (see inset) and palms shoulder width apart. Tuck your toes under, bend your legs, and lift your hips up toward the ceiling.

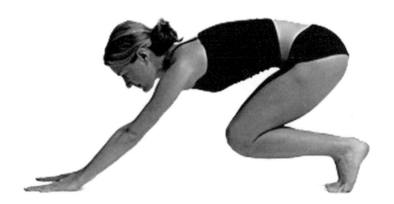

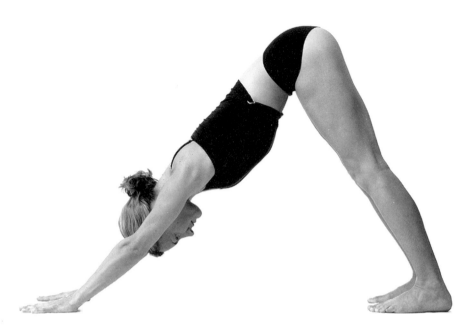

Press your fingers and palms firmly into the floor. Keep your spine straight and long, with your feet hip width apart and toes facing forward. Gently press your heels into the floor as you lift your butt up and start to straighten your legs. Feel the stretch in the backs of your legs. If necessary, you can bend your legs to keep your back straight. Over time your legs should become straight. Pull your thigh muscles up and gaze just above your kneecaps, lengthening your neck. Now squeeze your lower abs and sexual core in and up toward the sky, as if to touch your spine with your belly button. Take your weight off your arms and legs by visualizing a thick strap around your hip bones drawing you up toward the ceiling. Breathe deeply all the way into your pubic bone and expand everywhere! Hold for five breaths. To release, bend your knees and lower yourself back into On All Fours. To fully relax, come all the way down to Chill Out (page 60).

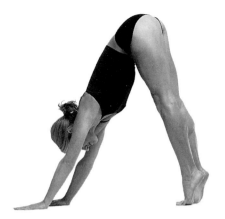

For a deep sexy stretch, lift your heels high off the floor, tilt your pelvis forward, and lift your tailbone up. Flex and pull the tops of your thigh muscles up toward your hips. Deepen the pose by raising your heels higher, lifting your butt higher, and walking your hands closer to your feet. Slowly release your heels to the floor with your butt in the air. Repeat three times. Experimenting with this position will give you greater mobility and greater pleasure during the Oops, I Dropped the Soap! sex position.

CHAKRAS 1 to 7

HOTTIE BODY		**IN THE BEDROOM**	
· long, lean legs		· Doggie Style	
· sexy shoulders and arms		· Double Triangle	
· supple spine		· Oops, I Dropped the Soap!	
· wrinkle reducer		· Rock Steady	
· healthy hair		· Surf's Up	

hot tip { Roll your shoulder blades to the outside toward your pinkies and flex your feet so your heels move closer to the floor. Feel your breath go so deeply that it expands your lower back and pelvis. Push back into this position as a "breather" when you are a top dog in Surf's Up. If your man is on top, this is a great reliever to help him last longer.

WARRIOR I

This pose is a total body energizer. By mastering this pose, you'll strengthen your legs, open your hips, and tone your tummy. Warrior I also improves concentration and balance as well as circulation and respiration.

TO DO IT

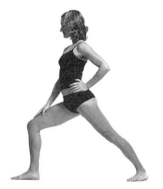

From an upright standing position, step forward with your right foot into a lunge, keeping your feet hip width apart and facing forward. Keep your right knee directly over your right ankle. Put your hands on your hips, and make sure your hips and shoulders are square to the wall in front of you.

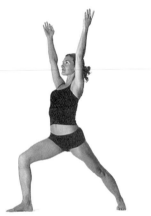

Bring your arms over your head alongside the front of your ears with your palms facing each other. Drop your shoulders down and back, and expand your chest. Breathe in and out of your lower back and pelvis five times. To release, straighten your front knee and step forward into a standing upright position. Repeat on the other side.

VARIATIONS

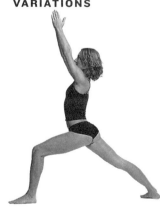

PALMS TOGETHER

Touch your palms together with your arms straight and above your head. Be sure to keep your shoulders low and your shoulder blades squeezed together.

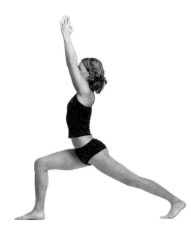

CRESCENT

Do the same as in Palms Together, only balance on the ball of your back foot, with both hips facing forward.

CHAKRAS 1, 3, 4, 5

HOTTIE BODY
- yoga butt
- sexy shoulders
- toned lats
- long, lean legs

IN THE BEDROOM
- Bridging the Gap
- The Conquest
- Satisfying Side
- Surf's Up

hot tip { To get the most out of this pose, make sure that your tailbone is facing down, your spine is straight, and your pelvis is tucked under. The outside edge of your back foot should be pressing into the floor with the same pressure as the inside of your foot. Your back leg should be completely straight, thigh muscle lifted from the knee. This empowering and authoritative pose will bring you confidence to experiment with your partner.

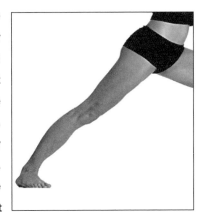

CRAVE

Aptly named, this hybrid position leaves you wanting more sex. You crave a beautiful body, and this pose will get you there. Once you master this pose, expect a flatter tummy, a gorgeous butt, strong arms and legs, and the grace of a dancer.

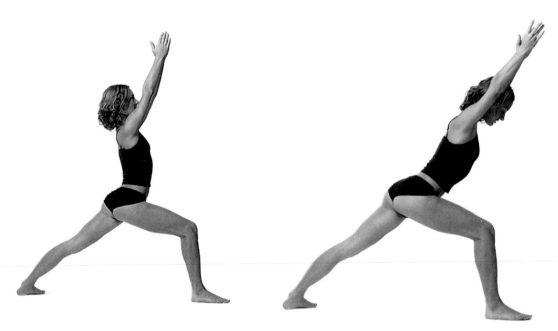

TO DO IT Starting in Warrior I (page 134), tilt forward at the waist so that you are making a diagonal line from the tips of your fingers to the end of your backmost heel. Keep your shoulders away from your ears and your arms straight up by your ears. Then look down toward your big toe, keeping your neck in line with your spine, and lengthen your torso by reaching your chest forward. Be sure to keep your jaw and mouth loose. Hold here for four full breaths.

CHAKRAS 1, 2, 4, 7

HOTTIE BODY
· yummy tummy
· flexible back
· strong and toned arms and legs

IN THE BEDROOM
· Backseat Buddies
· Oops, I Dropped the Soap!
· Surf's Up
· Talking in Tongues

hot tip { Practicing this pose will help to both strengthen and relax your neck, allowing for more grace during fellatio. You'll be dying to show off in the bedroom.

WARRIOR II

As invigorating as Warrior I, Warrior II strengthens the lower body and arms; stretches the groin, chest, lungs, and shoulders; and increases stamina. It is also a great pose for the guy in your life because it stretches and strengthens his prostate.

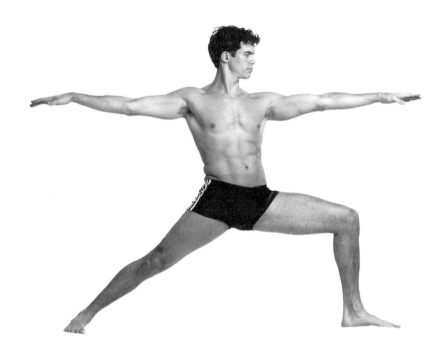

TO DO IT From Warrior I (page 134), inhale deeply and rise up slightly as you turn your hips to face the left side of the room. Exhale and gracefully lower your arms so that they are parallel to the floor. Turn your left foot in the same direction as your left hand, and bend your left knee directly over your left ankle in a mock lunge. Turn and look beyond the left middle finger. Keep your legs strong and steady. Relax your hips, allowing them to sink toward the floor (feel the flex in your left inner thigh), and stretch the crown of your head up to the ceiling. Relax your shoulders and open your chest. Breathe deeply five times.

CHAKRAS 1, 4, 5, 6, 7

HOTTIE BODY
- yoga butt
- great legs
- calm and serene face
- supple arms

IN THE BEDROOM
- Rock Steady
- Splitting Bamboo

hot tip { Your tailbone should be pointed down at the floor and tucked under your spine. Lift the crown of the head to the ceiling. Keep your upper body floating lightly above your strong and grounded legs to get energy flowing in your sexual core.

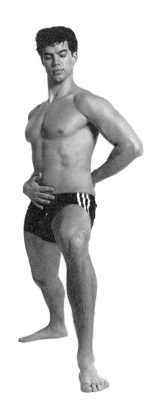

OPEN WIDE
This pose tones your abs, lengthens your spinal column, and stretches the backs of your legs and back muscles. It also focuses your attention on the pelvis so that you can experience what the tiniest tilt forward can do for you during sex.

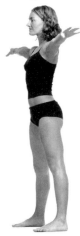

TO DO IT Stand with your legs open wide (about three or four feet), your arms straight out at your sides at shoulder height, and your head looking forward.

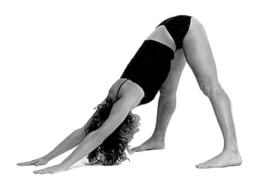

Angle your feet inward slightly and bend forward, leading with your chin and chest. Touch the floor and slide your hands out in front of you. Relax your head and neck between your shoulders. Lift your hips toward the ceiling, feeling an intense stretch in the backs of your legs. As in Downward Dog (page 130), tilt your pelvis forward and stretch the tailbone toward the ceiling.

This tilt will elongate the space between your navel and pubic bone and straighten your lower back. Remain here and breathe deeply into your pelvic core five times. Practice tilting your pelvis in the opposite direction, to tuck the tailbone under, by squeezing your belly button toward your spine. To release, bend both knees, place your hands on your thighs, and slowly roll up.

VARIATION

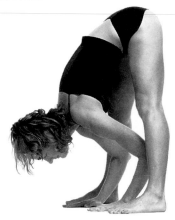

Place your hands directly beneath you. Line up your fingers with your toes and lower your face toward the floor. Keep your elbows bent and squeezed together so that your forearms are parallel to each other. Keep your chin lifted and your neck long. Practice the pelvic tilt, as you did in the regular pose. Remain here for five full breaths. Breathe deeply into your pelvic core.

CHAKRAS 1, 2, 3, 4, 5

HOTTIE BODY
- yoga butt
- defined and glorious glutes
- sexy lower lumbar curve

IN THE BEDROOM
- Backward-Forward Bend
- Double Triangle
- Oops, I Dropped the Soap!
- Splitting Bamboo

hot tip { Try stretching your feet by lifting your toes into the air with the soles of your feet flat on the floor. To get the ultimate sexual benefits of pelvic tilting, keep your legs taut and firm with your thigh muscles lifted from the knee to the groin.

HELLO

This mid-back twist position is a great stretch for the back of the legs and also increases strength in the sexual core and hips.

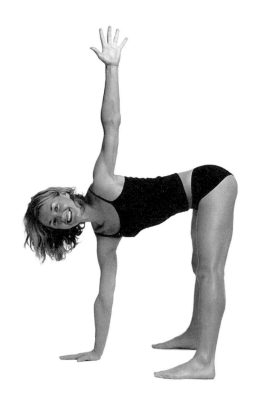

TO DO IT Stand with your legs wide open (about three feet apart) with your feet pointed directly forward. Bend at the waist and touch your hands to the floor, moving them forward so that your back is straight in a relaxed position. Place your right hand directly under your chin, then swing your left arm up toward the ceiling. Gaze down or toward the left side of the room with your neck long. Hold for four deep breaths. Repeat on the other side.

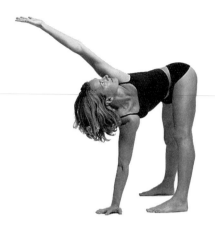

LOOSE HELLO

This is a free-form position, so do what feels best for you. You do this pose in the same way as Hello, but now stretch your left arm up over your head as far as you can while releasing neck tension. Try moving right hand on the floor toward your left foot, and play with this hand position to find any tight spots.

CHAKRAS 1, 2, 3, 7

HOTTIE BODY
- yoga butt
- tight triceps
- yummy tummy
- whittled waistline
- shapely shoulders

IN THE BEDROOM
- Doggie Style
- Double Triangle
- Oops, I Dropped the Soap!
- Satisfying Side

hot tip { Keep in mind that this is a mid-back twist, so keep your hips "square," or parallel, to the floor and resist the tendency to lift one hip. Your partner will appreciate this the next time you try Doggie Style in bed!

143

MODERN BREATH

This is a sexy and energizing move created to open your whole body through focused breathing. It does a great job of releasing back, shoulder, chest, and pelvic tension while stimulating energy in the heart, kidney, and spleen.

TO DO IT

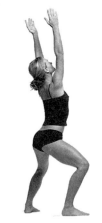

Stand with your legs open wide. Inhale deeply, raising both arms above your head.

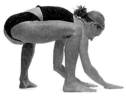

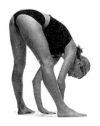

Exhale deeply, arching your back, bending your knees, and lowering your arms—leading with the forearms—to the floor in between your feet.

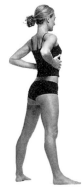

Inhale and straighten your legs, and sexily drag your hands up the front of your body, running your fingers over any tense areas. Finish with your arms above your head.

CHAKRAS 1, 2, 4, 7

HOTTIE BODY
- yoga butt
- flexible lower back
- long, lean legs
- loose hips
- open chest

IN THE BEDROOM
- Bridging the Gap
- The Conquest
- Oops, I Dropped the Soap!
- Yin Yang

hot tip { Try running your hands up the sides of your body, exploring your sexy curvaceous waist. This will make the move even hotter.

HIP-HOP BOOTIE

Borrowed from a hip-hop class, this booty-licious move is sure to grab your partner's attention. This pose is especially naughty if he's watching from behind during a peep show. It will get you both in the mood and keep foreplay light and playful.

TO DO IT

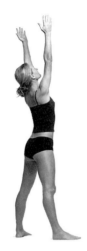

Stand with your legs wide apart (about three feet). Inhale deeply, raising both arms above your head. Keep your arms straight above your head.

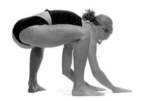

Bend your legs so that your thighs are parallel to the floor and your hands are resting on the floor in front of you.

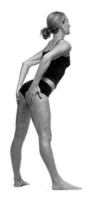

Stand up so that your torso is leaning forward. Reach back and place your hands on your butt.

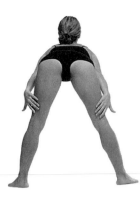

Lean completely forward so that your back is now parallel to the floor. Run your hands down your legs. (This should feel sexy.)

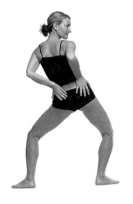

Now look behind you, bend your knees, and rock twice—little bumps—to one side. Strike a pose, and repeat on the other side.

CHAKRAS 2, 5

HOTTIE BODY
· yoga butt
· fabulous face
· healthy hair
· long, lean legs

IN THE BEDROOM
· Oops, I Dropped the Soap!
· Rearview
· Splitting Bamboo
· Talking in Tongues

hot tip { Lighten up! This is a fun pose. Let go of what you think you should look like and do what feels good to you. Trust us, that's when your partner will find you sexiest.

HULA HIPS

A fun and groovy pose, Hula Hips adds a little swerve into your yoga flow while improving your pelvic flexibility. It's a super way to shake out your back after a long day of work.

TO DO IT

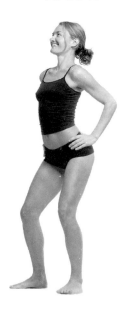

Stand with your feet about three feet apart, with your knees slightly bent and your chest slightly puffed out.

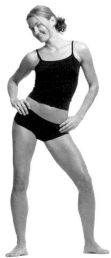

Put your hands on the sides of your waist, fingers in front and thumbs in the back, and move your hips forward, right, back, then left. As you move your hips forward, inhale and contract your PC muscles; as you move backward, exhale and release your PC muscles. Once you get the hang of it, loosen up! Put your shoulders and chest into it, and swivel your hips clockwise, taking about three seconds to complete each circuit.

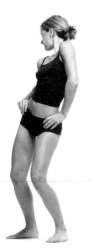

Arch your back and push your chest forward, move your hips to one side curving your waistline, then tuck your tailbone under and around your back. Move in smooth, continuous circles ten times, then reverse and move counterclockwise ten times.

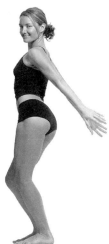

Raise your arms from your hips and swing them to match your moves. Go for it and swing them in any way that feels good!

CHAKRAS 1, 2, 3

HOTTIE BODY	· whittled waist

IN THE BEDROOM	· Oops, I Dropped the Soap!
	· Satisfying Side
	· Wild Child

hot tip { Keep your feet flat on the floor and really work those hips. Swiveling your hips while squatting over your man while he is seated or lying down will get you both really hot, really fast.

TRIANGLE
The Triangle pose engages every part of your body, strengthens your sexual core, opens your hips and shoulders, as well as stretches your groin, hamstrings, hips, and calves. It also helps relieve stress and anxiety. Remember, stress is one of the biggest sex busters.

TO DO IT

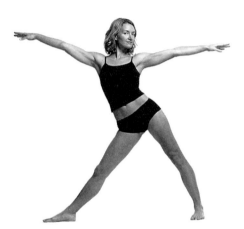

From a standing upright position, open your legs wide (about three feet). Turn your right toes toward the right wall and your left foot 45 degrees inward. Bring your arms up parallel to the floor. First rock your hips to the left, then to the right, then back to the left and hold. Loosen up those hips!

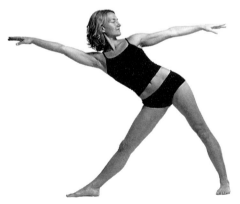

Look at your left hand while tilting over to the right side, resting your right hand against your right shin. Make sure to pull your thigh muscles up from the knee. Bend your front knee slightly to prevent hyperextending. Reach your fingertips away from each other, bringing your arms into one straight line. Actively use your oblique and abdominal muscles to lift toward the ceiling. Do not sink into your right hip. Breathe deeply five times, then release. Inhale and stand up. Repeat on the other side.

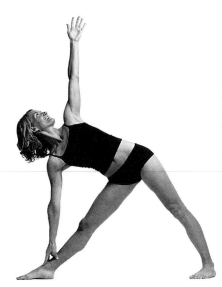

Instead of putting your hand on your shin, put your hand on your ankle or foot. For an even deeper stretch, wrap your index and middle fingers around your big toe. Push the toe down and pull up from the waist.

CHAKRAS 2, 3, 4

HOTTIE BODY	· whittled waistline · drop-dead abs

IN THE BEDROOM	· The Conquest · Double Triangle · Splitting Bamboo

hot tip { Keep your neck long and sexy. Find your balance through a lifted inner core. Add the hip rock for a more flexible pelvis and to look like a real pro in bed.

BENT-KNEE TRIANGLE

This leg-strengthening posture will define your inner thighs while sculpting your oblique muscles (on the sides of your waist). This pose also encourages you to "open your heart" as you gently twist your torso.

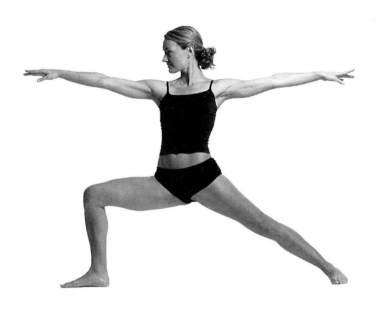

TO DO IT Begin as you would in Warrior II (page 138) with your legs open wide, right knee bent, back leg straight, and your arms shoulder height.

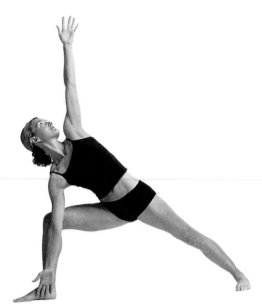

Gaze beyond your right hand and extend from your waist. Without changing your leg positions, tilt at the waist and lightly touch your inner ankle with the backs of your right fingers. Reach your left hand high up toward the ceiling and hold. Ideally, you should form a straight line from your left armpit to the edge of your left heel. Repeat on the other side.

CHAKRAS 1, 2, 4, 7

HOTTIE BODY
- yoga butt
- long and strong legs
- sexy shoulders

IN THE BEDROOM
- Backseat Buddies
- Double Triangle

hot tip
Be sure to keep your back foot flat on the floor and your tailbone pointing down. The hip opening and inner thigh strengthening will allow you to spread your legs wider and straddle your man more easily than you ever imagined. It will keep him coming back for more. We promise.

REVERSE TRIANGLE
This pose will help you to stretch out your hamstrings and mid-back, tone your abdomen, and prepare you for the Double Triangle sex pose with your honey. If that's not enough incentive, this pose also aids in digestion and eliminates excess gas. Unexpected gas can be a real mood spoiler.

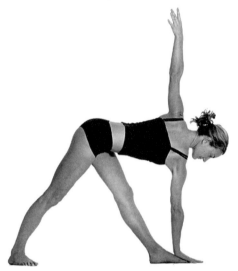

TO DO IT

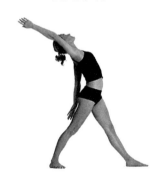

Stand with your legs wide apart (about three feet), your left leg in front of your right. Your back foot should be on an angle, and your hips squared directly forward. (Give your hips a few gentle twists and be sure you are facing straight ahead.) Lift your right arm above your head, and keep your left arm low and by your side. Look up and bend back, giving your back a nice stretch.

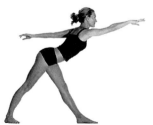

Stretch your right arm forward, making a straight line from your tailbone to your fingertips, while reaching your left hand behind you. Lean forward and reach your right arm as far as you can (until your back is flat).

154

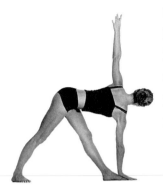

Lower your right hand to the top of your foot or shin and raise your left arm toward the ceiling, bringing your arms into a straight line. Keep your lower back flat and your hips parallel to the floor, then turn your head to the right and look straight ahead. Be sure to keep your neck long. Hold for five deep breaths. To release, look down at your lower hand, then stand up. Repeat on the other side.

CHAKRAS 2, 3, 5

HOTTIE BODY
· long, lean legs
· whittled waist
· sexy shoulders and arms
· yummy tummy
· yoga butt

IN THE BEDROOM
· Backward-Forward Bend
· Double Triangle
· Splitting Bamboo

hot tip { Once in the pose, lengthen the space between your tailbone and the top of your head by squeezing through your sexual core. Try squeezing your vaginal walls to make this a really "tight fit" for your partner.

SIDE ANGLE
This delicious move lets you stretch and tone the sides of your torso, obliques, and abs. It nicely opens the hips and defines your quads. The subtle upper-body twist encourages an open heart and deep breathing.

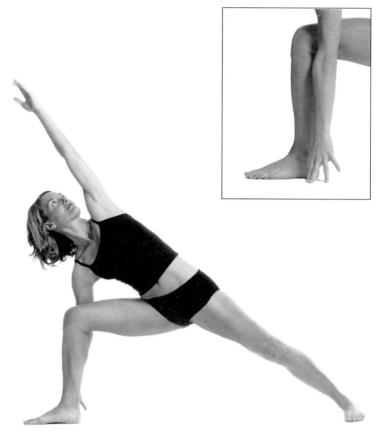

TO DO IT Begin in Downward Dog (page 130). Inhale and step your right leg up in between your hands. At the same time, drop your back heel to touch the floor and reach your left arm up over your head, close to your left ear. Keep your right hand at the side of your right ankle, with only the tips of your fingers on the floor (see inset). Keep no weight on this hand! Gaze under your left elbow at the ceiling and hold for five full breaths. Exhale and return to Downward Dog. Repeat on the other side.

CHAKRAS 2, 3, 4, 5

HOTTIE BODY
- yoga butt
- yummy tummy
- luscious lats
- tight triceps

IN THE BEDROOM
- The Conquest
- Rock Steady
- Surf's Up

hot tip { For drop-dead abs that make your partner beg for more, use your stomach muscles to twist your body sideways from the waist. This also makes gazing under your elbow a cinch.

HALF MOON

This is a great pose if you like to have sex standing up. (Okay, admit it—you like to stand up and do it once in a while.) It really builds power in the thighs while stretching out your groin.

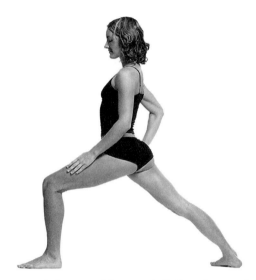

TO DO IT Stand in a mock lunge with your left foot forward and your right leg back, foot angled in.

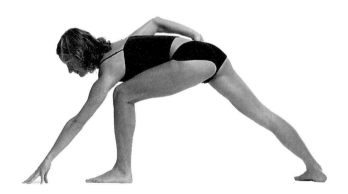

Place your right hand on your hip, bend your left knee, and place your left hand on the floor a couple of inches in front and *slightly* to the outside of your toes.

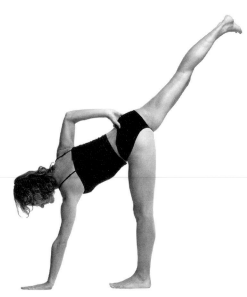

Inhale, push off of your back leg, and come to balance on your left hand and left leg. Twist your right shoulder by moving your elbow behind your back. Flex your right foot and push your heel up behind you. Squeeze your left butt and glutes and lift your leg as high as you can. Hold for five full breaths. Repeat on the other side.

CHAKRAS 1, 2, 4, 6

HOTTIE BODY
· yoga butt
· long and strong legs
· whittled waist
· yummy tummy

IN THE BEDROOM
· Satisfying Side
· Splitting Bamboo

hot tip {
Be sure to line your back leg directly behind you so that your heel lines up with your tailbone to improve overall flexibility. Do not cross your leg over; doing so will twist your spine. When you are flexible enough to get your back leg pretty high, have your partner hold your hips and enter you from behind. See if you can remain in the pose, and then try placing your hand on the floor for better balance.

NECK AND SHOULDER RELEASE *This is one of the quickest and easiest do-anywhere stretches for releasing neck and shoulder tension. This move also tones your heart and pericardium (the protective wrapper around your heart) and improves your lung energy. Remember, these are all good things for lovin'.*

TO DO IT

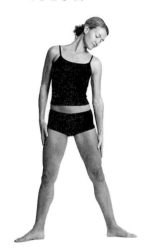

Standing with your feet slightly wider than hip width apart, gently lower your left ear toward your left shoulder, then your right ear toward your right shoulder. Move your head back to the left and circle forward with your chin to your chest. Feel a nice stretch at the back of your neck, then circle to the right and come up.

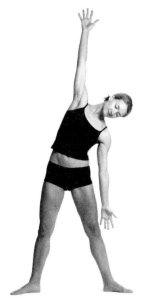

Raise your right arm toward the ceiling and stretch your left arm down toward the floor.

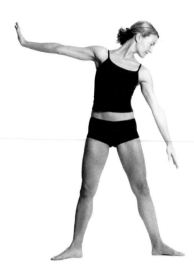

Lower your right arm so that it's parallel to the floor with your hand flexed back. Stretch your left arm toward the floor. Turn and look over your left shoulder for an exquisite stretch through the whole arm, shoulder, and neck. Repeat the entire sequence on the other side.

CHAKRAS 4, 5

HOTTIE BODY	· sexy shoulders
	· relaxed neck
	· radiant face
	· open chest

IN THE BEDROOM	· Bathing Beauties
	· Orgasmic Camel
	· Satisfying Side
	· Talking in Tongues

hot tip { This is such an important stretch we repeat it in our "Sexy Secretary" section. Doing this stretch with regularity will help keep neck, arm, and carpal pain away and also keep you loose in bed. We also love this as a warm-up pose because it's great for flexing your neck for better kissing.

DANCING BEAUTY

This modern dance stretch nicely loosens the shoulders, hamstrings, and spine. It also really adds grace to your routine and gives you a unique, sexy style.

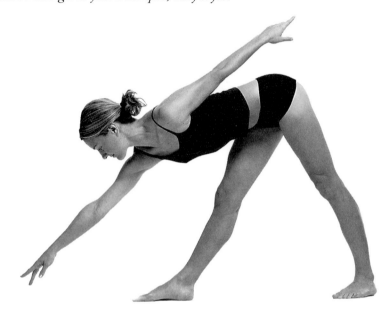

TO DO IT

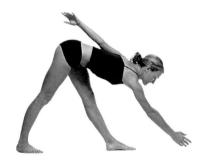

Stand with your legs open about two feet. Bending at the waist, reach your right arm across your chest, then sweep out and down and touch the floor, stretching out the hamstrings.

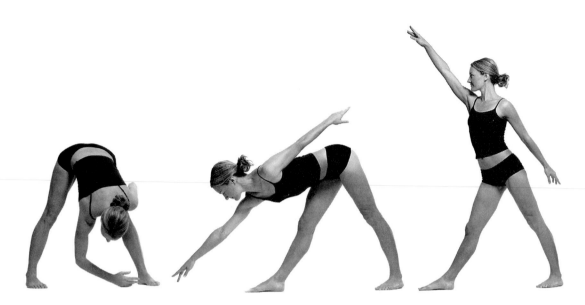

Lean over to your right side and circle forward. Let your arms dangle, keeping your neck relaxed and your shoulders loose. Use your whole body to circle back up.

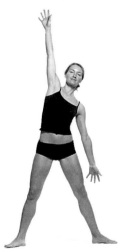

Reach your right arm straight up to the ceiling and your left arm straight down to the floor. Hold and stretch.

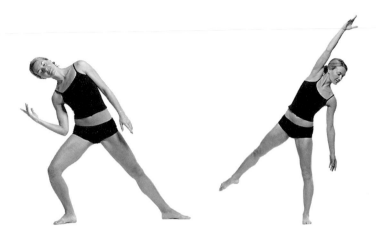

Facing forward, bend your right knee and right elbow, then straighten both legs and throw your right arm high up and over your head. Keep your left arm by your side.

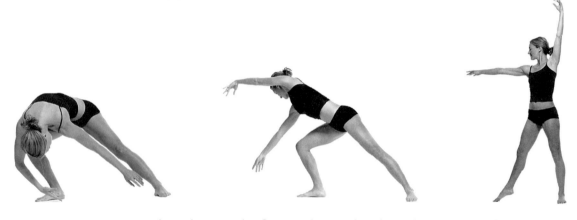

Circle and sweep the floor with your hands, ending in a standing position with your right arm straight out to the right and your left arm reaching up. Repeat on the other side.

CHAKRAS 2, 3, 4, 6, 7

HOTTIE
BODY
- whittled waistline
- yummy tummy
- yoga butt
- sexy and relaxed neck
- long, lean legs

_____

IN THE
BEDROOM
- Backseat Buddies
- Oops, I Dropped the Soap!

hot tip **{** Remember to always keep your abdomen lifted and your breathing full and deep for ultimate satisfaction.

STANDING FORWARD BEND

A great anxiety and fatigue fighter, this pose lengthens your spine and stretches the back of your legs and back muscles while stimulating your digestive and nervous systems. This pose also brings energy and blood to the head, providing you with healthy, shiny hair, emotional stability, and greater energy.

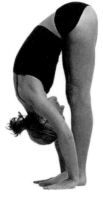

TO DO IT

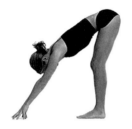

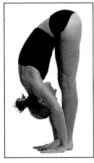

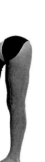

Stand with your feet touching, bend forward with a flat back by creating a "hinge" between your upper body and legs. If necessary, bend your knees so you can place your hands on the floor. Feel free to walk your hands as far forward as necessary to touch the floor, elongating your spine.

Focus on keeping your stomach hollowed out and your neck and shoulders relaxed. Having your hands out in front of you makes it easier not only to reach the floor but also to feel your abdominal muscles engaging. Once you've figured out how much body weight your core muscles can hold, work your hands closer to the sides of your feet and press your nose to your knees, if you can (see inset). Move your hands as close to your feet as your core muscles can withstand while supporting your upper body weight. Feel the top of your spine and tailbone stretching in opposite directions. Relax your neck, and face your knees or shins with hips lifting toward the ceiling. Breathe deeply in the pose five times. To release, keep your back straight, squeeze your legs together, and inhale while returning to standing position.

166

VARIATION (INTERMEDIATE) Cup your fingers under your heels so that your palms are pressed against your heels and your fingers are under the arches of your feet.

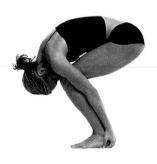 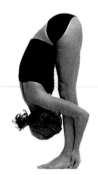

Pull your torso close to your legs.

VARIATION (ADVANCED)

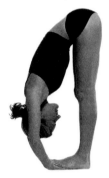

Cup your fingers under your toes and walk the balls of your feet to your arms. Again, use your arm strength and pull your torso close to your legs.

CHAKRAS 1, 2, 7

HOTTIE BODY	**IN THE BEDROOM**
· whittled waistline	· Backward-Forward Bend
· glorious glutes	· Doggie Style
· long, lean legs	· Oops, I Dropped the Soap!
· supple spine	· Rearview
· flexible lower back	

hot tip { This position takes and makes great arm strength. Don't forget to pull your upper body close to your legs and relax your neck for strong arms that can help you do more in the bedroom.

167

CANDY CANE
This pose helps to increase concentration, mental focus, and balance while toning your inner core and butt.

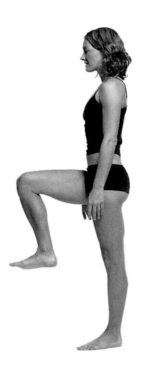

TO DO IT In a standing position, shift your weight to one side and raise your opposite knee so that your thigh is parallel to the floor and your foot is flexed.

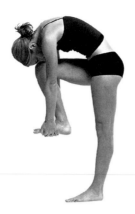

From the waist, curl forward like a giant candy cane, touching your forehead to your knee and placing your hands underneath your foot. Your balance should come from your abdominal strength; don't put too much weight onto your hands. Stare at one point on the floor and calm your mind to keep balanced. Try to keep your standing leg straight with your muscles taut. Breathe deeply five times. To release, slowly let go of your bent leg and return to an upright standing position. Repeat on the other side.

CHAKRAS 2, 3, 6

HOTTIE BODY
- yummy tummy
- yoga butt
- defined calf muscles

IN THE BEDROOM
- The Conquest
- Rock Steady
- Splitting Bamboo
- Talking in Tongues

hot tip { Keep your stomach tight and feel the lift in your sexual core. Try to keep your standing leg straight and strong with your thigh muscle and kneecap pulling upward. Do not lock your knees.

STANDING BEAU

This pose improves balance, focus, and concentration while stretching and strengthening your hips, legs, back, and shoulders. Best of all, it reduces that loose abdominal fat for sexy abs and a sexy you in the bedroom.

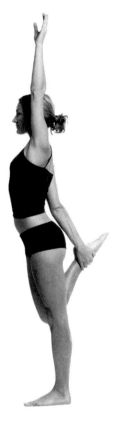

TO DO IT Starting from an upright standing position, raise your left hand toward the ceiling. Shift your weight to your left foot and bend the right knee. Reach back with your right hand and hold the inside of the right foot. Point your right foot and bring your knees close together.

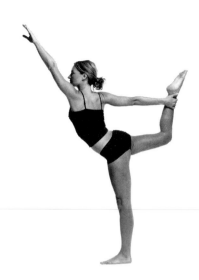

Inhale deeply, reach up to the ceiling, and on an exhale, tilt forward, bringing your left arm to forehead level. At the same time push back strongly with your right leg and pull with your right arm. Keep your chin and chest lifted and look out and over your left fingertips. Keep your right hip down, parallel to the floor. Breathe in and out of your sexual core five times. To release, inhale and reach up one more inch before returning to standing, touching your knees together and lowering your foot and arm. Repeat on the other side.

CHAKRAS 1 to 7

HOTTIE BODY
- yoga butt
- yummy tummy
- open chest

IN THE BEDROOM
- Doggie Style
- Erotic Froggie
- Oops, I Dropped the Soap!
- Orgasmic Camel

hot tip { If flexibility comes easy for you, instead of holding the inside of your foot, try holding near or above the ankle. This ensures extension in your chest and back. If you're into multitasking during sex, this could be fun for both receiving and giving oral sex. Try kicking back your leg and leaning over the bed to do Talking in Tongues.

CUPID'S ARROW

This balancing posture builds concentration for that stay-in-the-moment focus. It also tones and invigorates your sexual core by connecting your lower back with your abs and inner thighs while increasing blood flow to your heart.

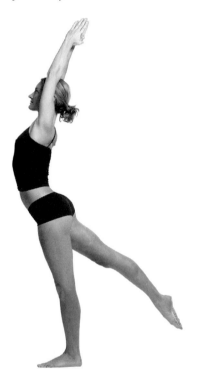

TO DO IT From a standing upright position, raise your arms up over your head and clasp your hands. Draw your elbows back behind your ears. Step forward onto your left foot, raise your right leg off the floor behind you, and point your toes.

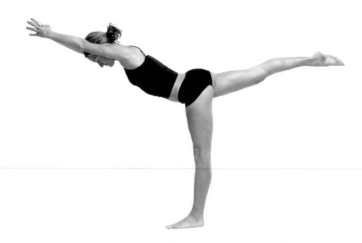

Take a deep breath, then exhale and tilt forward, bringing your arms, torso, and right leg parallel to the floor. Look down at the floor and stare at a point just ahead of your big toe for balance. Breathe deeply in and out into your sexual core five times. Then release, inhale, and lower your elevated leg back to the floor to return to a standing upright position. Lower your arms to your sides and repeat on other side.

CHAKRAS 1, 2, 5

HOTTIE BODY
- flexible lower back
- sexy shoulders
- yoga butt
- open chest
- long, lean legs

IN THE BEDROOM
- The Conquest
- Satisfying Side
- Yin Yang

hot tip { Squeeze your legs, particularly noticing the thigh muscles as you lift up off your standing leg. Don't drop onto your hip. Squeeze your glutes too to help define that yoga butt.

TREE *This pose increases balance, focus, memory, and concentration while strengthening your ankles and knees, tightening your glutes and thighs, and opening your groin and inner thighs.*

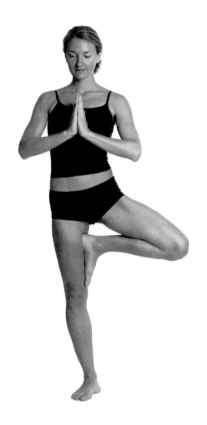

TO DO IT From a standing upright position, shift your weight to your right foot, bend and lift your left knee, and take hold of your left foot. Open your knee to the side and place the sole of your left foot on your right inner thigh, as high as comfortably possible. Look straight ahead and focus on one point for balance. When you are balanced here, slowly bring your palms together in a prayer position in front of your heart. Try not to grip the floor with your toes. Hold for five breaths. With each inhale, imagine your breath traveling down and into your sexual core from your heart. To release, slowly let go of your bent leg and return to a standing upright position. Repeat on the other side.

CHAKRAS 1, 2, 4

HOTTIE
BODY
· loose hips
· yoga butt
· dancer's posture
· supple knees

_____

IN THE
BEDROOM
· Erotic Froggie
· Rearview

hot tip { Be aware of your knees—this posture can stress them if you're not keeping your quads and glutes strong. This pose really stimulates your reproductive organs and energizes you so that having more sex won't tire you out.

DUO ASSISTED POSES

Are you ready to really head things up and push the limits of your comfort zone? Then these Duo Assisted Poses are for you and your partner to do together. Downward Dog by yourself is great, but when you've got a partner pushing into the stretch, you might just end up in Doggie Style like dogs in heat. It's been known to happen. We don't take responsibility for what happens after you practice any of these duo poses. Most people don't even make it to the next pose in the series and find themselves entangled in pleasure.

DUO DOWNWARD DOG *As with solo Downward Dog, this pose is great for stretching the hamstrings and calf muscles, loosening and lengthening your back, and freeing up your pelvis by loosening your hips.*

TO DO IT

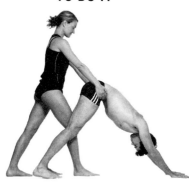

Assist your partner doing Downward Dog (page 130) by cupping your hands over his hip bones and gently pulling up. Be sure to stand close to your partner as you step your leg between his for leverage. Instruct your partner to keep reaching with his arms forward as you elongate his back. This is also a great opportunity to encourage your partner to breathe deeply into his lower back.

CHAKRAS All of them!

HOTTIE BODY
- sexy shoulders and arms
- long, lean legs
- loose hips

IN THE BEDROOM
- Oops, I Dropped the Soap!

hot tip { Not only will this loosen your partner's hamstrings, but it will enable the sexual core to have a greater range of motion.

DUO SEATED FORWARD BEND *This move seriously deepens your forward bend. Plus, the extra weight of your lover will easily take this stretch to a new level.*

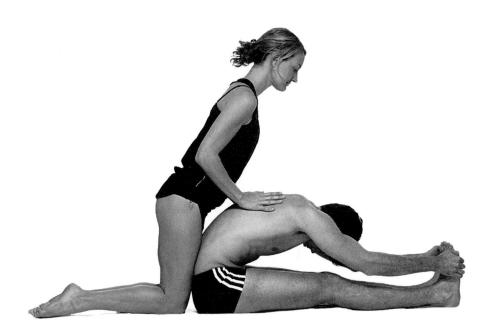

TO DO IT Kneel directly behind your partner with your thighs touching his back. Have him take hold of his feet and bend forward, lowering his chin to his chest. Begin to lower yourself over his back as you walk your hands up his back. You can use this moment to give his back and neck a quick massage.

Use all of your body weight and fully relax your neck. Reach forward and grab hold of your partner's feet, flexing his toes to straighten his legs. Encourage him to press his knees into the floor. Hold and breathe deeply into your lower back and sexual core. To release, walk your hands back down his back and kneel behind him. Make sure you come up slowly, as this deep hinge in your lower back can produce a serious head rush for you and your partner.

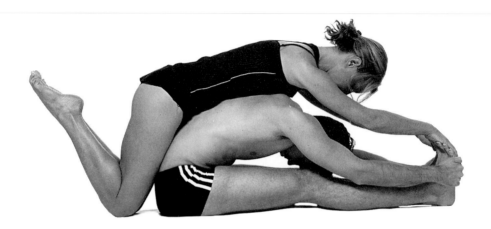

CHAKRAS 1, 2, 3

HOTTIE BODY
· supple spine
· loose hips
· sexy and stretchy hamstrings

IN THE BEDROOM
· Backward-Forward Bend
· Splitting Bamboo

hot tip { When assisting your lover, encourage deep breathing and apply more pressure only when your mate exhales. Use your body weight and relax—this ensures a safer and more comfortable assist (for both of you!). However, do listen and be patient with your partner if he's very tight (most guys are). Learning to communicate and understand your lover's body will make pillow talk during sex all the more meaningful.

DUO BUTTERFLY

Another great reason for full body contact—this one opens the hips and hits the nerves down there like no other! This pose counters the effects of sitting cramped at a desk or in a car all day. While opening your hips, it also nicely loosens your lower back and neck.

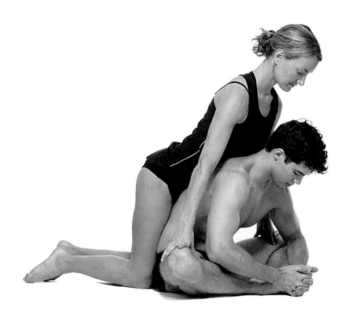

TO DO IT Start by kneeling at your partner's back, with your thighs pressing up to his back to prop it straight. Your partner either presses his thumbs into the ball of his feet to spread them open or clasps his feet and bends forward. At first, both of you should keep your backs straight and your necks long. Then, at the same time, lower your heads forward and curve your backs. Move your hands onto your partner's thighs and use your body's weight to push them closer to the floor.

Note: Some people have tight hips and can't take too much weight near their knees, so you might want to put more weight on his back instead. Communicating with your partner is always the best approach. Hold and breathe deeply four full breaths.

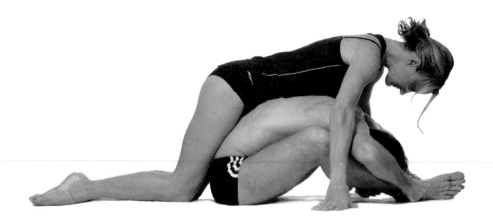

If your partner is not very flexible, have him extend his Butterfly by moving his feet farther out in front of him. To adjust, do the same as above, only lay your abdomen higher up on your partner's back and then relax forward, using your body weight to help him stretch. Place your hands on the floor just in front of his knees.

CHAKRAS 1, 2, 3

HOTTIE BODY
- killer inner thighs
- loose hips
- pliable pelvis

IN THE BEDROOM
- Rock Steady
- Talking in Tongues

hot tip { When adjusting your position, move your weight forward over your partner to deepen the stretch and heighten the intimacy of the pose. Let's face it, the greater intimacy between you and your partner, the better the sex.

DUNKING FOR APPLES
A variation on our In the Saddle, this pose will stretch your inner thighs to their limit. Pay close attention to your partner, and stretch his thighs only as far as they will go comfortably.

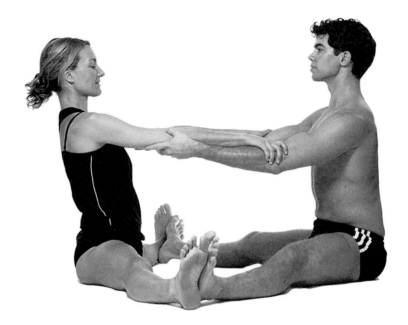

TO DO IT Begin by sitting on the floor in In the Saddle (page 96), with your feet touching and your backs straight. Take firm hold of each other's wrists or forearms. One at a time, bend forward, and attempt to keep your back nice and straight. (You may need to make adjustments if you and your partner are at different flexibility levels.)

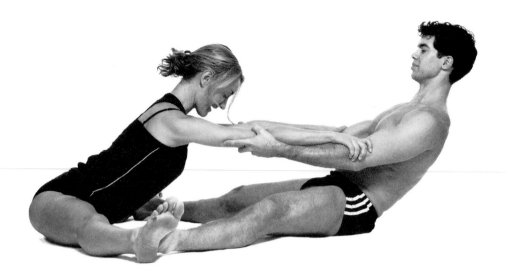

Your legs can be wider (like Jacquie), and you may bend your back and lower your head if you cannot maintain a flat back. Wherever you are in your practice, hold your partner tight, lean back, and give him a delicious and deep inner thigh stretch.

CHAKRAS 1, 2, 4

HOTTIE BODY
· killer inner thighs
· perfect posture

IN THE BEDROOM
· Erotic Froggie
· Rearview

hot tip { A note of caution: Gazing into each other's eyes with your genitals facing each other might distract you from ever getting to the next pose.

DOUBLE BOAT

Double your pleasure by doing the Boat to-gether. This is an unbelievable strength builder for your abs and quadriceps. The Double Boat lets you watch your partner as you each balance your sexual energies together.

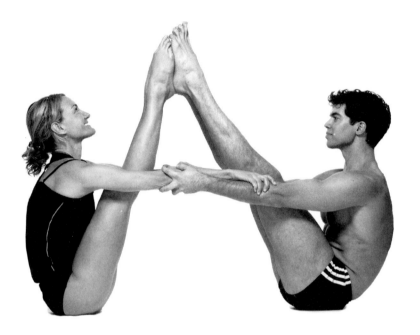

TO DO IT Sit on the floor facing each other with your knees bent, and hold on to each other's elbows or forearms. Touch the soles of your feet together and lift one leg at a time into Boat (page 118). Point your toes, try your best to keep your backs straight, and balance on your sit bones. Tighten and contract your abs, to better balance. Hold for two breaths, or for as long as your can.

CHAKRAS 2, 3, 6

HOTTIE BODY
- yummy tummy
- strong and sexy arms
- flexible back
- strong quads

———————

IN THE BEDROOM
- Backseat Buddies
- Backward-Forward Bend
- Splitting Bamboo

hot tip { This double balance pose takes a lot of control, flexibility, and patience, as you use your abs for balance and to keep your back straight. Achieving this pose requires focus and teamwork, which helps you and your partner connect both physically and emotionally.

DUO CAMEL

The best way to master the Orgasmic Camel is to have a little help. This pose is a breeze for the assistant yet a blessing for your yogi partner. It will gently stretch the chest and free up the flow of sexual energy in the lower abdomen.

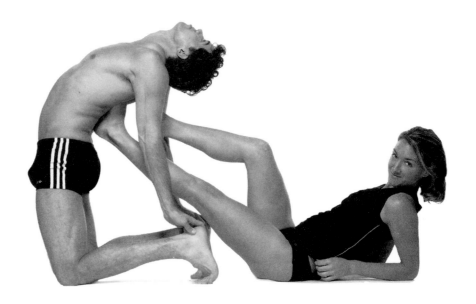

TO DO IT Lie down behind your partner as he bends backward into a Camel (page 62). Lightly place your feet on his back, one in the mid-back and one in between the shoulder blades. (Be sure to place your feet on the muscles on either sides of the spine and *never* directly on the bones or spine.) Gently push him forward while encouraging him to take his back bend farther. This assist will help him to let go completely, knowing you have his "back" covered. Have him hold for four deep breaths, then have him gently push up with your assistance.

CHAKRAS 2, 4, 5

HOTTIE BODY
- yummy tummy
- flexible back
- open chest and heart

IN THE BEDROOM
- Mermaid
- Orgasmic Camel
- Yin Yang

hot tip { This pose might be quite an intense experience, so be sure to give a Duo Chill Out with Massage (page 188) once he's out of the pose. What better way to transition into sex than with some massage as foreplay?

DUO CHILL OUT WITH MASSAGE *This assisted pose gives a great back stretch and is good to do after some of the tougher positions and also at the end of a yoga practice. It also stabilizes your partner's energy through acupressure, balancing, and massage.*

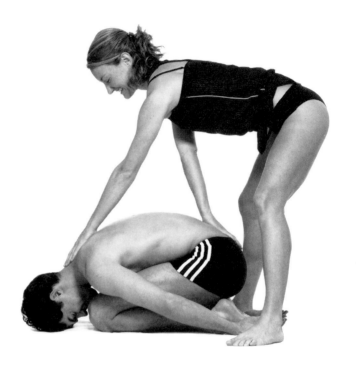

TO DO IT Stand behind your partner as he moves into Chill Out pose (page 60). Place one hand below the nape of his neck (at the top of his back, on the spine) and the other hand on top of the sacrum (his lower back). Press down, using your body weight, and press him deeper into the pose. Put a bit more weight on his sacrum, to help loosen up his hips. Then kneed the muscles in his lower back, using your fingertips for more direct pressure or your palms for a softer touch. Healthy, unkinked muscles of the lower back keep sexual energy potent.

CHAKRAS 2, 3, 4, 7

HOTTIE BODY
- radiant face
- wrinkle remover
- yummy tummy

IN THE BEDROOM
- Backward-Forward Bend
- Bundled Package

hot tip { Massage your partner whenever possible. It will bring you both pleasure and make for a happier, healthier, and more sexually tuned-in mate.

SEXY SECRETARY POSES

We know that sometimes squeezing sex, much less exercise, into your busy schedule can feel like a chore. We don't want either one to be squeezed out of your life. That's why we've incorporated these Sexy Secretary poses with the working girl in mind—the kind who's on the go 24/7. You can incorporate these poses into your workday to invigorate your body and mind. Most important, by the end of the day you'll be craving more, not less, sex. Getting in the mood, we know, is half the battle to great sex.

UPHOLDING HEAVEN
This pose draws energy from the heavens and earth to revitalize the whole body, particularly the chest, lungs, and heart. It is very grounding and helps focus you in the moment.

TO DO IT

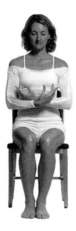

Stand or sit in perfect posture with your hands crossed at the wrists in front of your chest. Your knees should have a slight bend with your feet firmly planted on the floor.

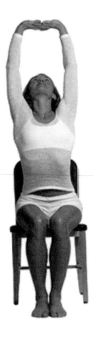

Inhale, raise both arms above the head, interlace your fingers, and reach up to the sky. Look up and inhale completely. Exhale and slowly lower your arms, returning them to a crossed position in front of your chest. Synchronize your breath with each movement.

CHAKRAS 1, 4, 7

HOTTIE BODY
- relaxed neck
- sexy shoulders
- loose wrists
- open heart

IN THE BEDROOM
- Bathing Beauties
- Wild Child
- Yin Yang

hot tip { When you inhale, make sure to inhale to the maximum. A big deep breath is a great way to release tension and keep you energized for the rest of your day (which we hope includes a romp in the sack with your partner).

NECK AND SHOULDER RELEASE (Sexy Secretary Version) *This is one of the quickest and easiest do-anywhere stretches for releasing neck and shoulder tension.*

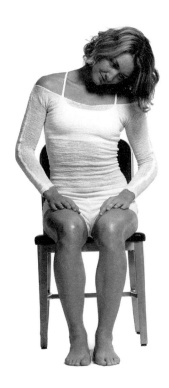

TO DO IT Begin by sitting in perfect posture with your hands in your lap. Gently lower your head to the left, then lower your head to the right. Move your head back to the left and circle forward with your chin to your chest. Repeat the circle and pause, holding your ear to your left shoulder.

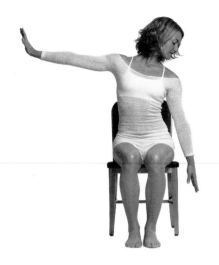

Raise your right arm and hold it at shoulder height, parallel to the floor, while flexing your fingers to the ceiling and pressing your palm outward, toward the side of the room. Turn and look over your opposite shoulder for an exquisite stretch through the whole arm, shoulder, and neck. Repeat the entire sequence to the other side, beginning with your head to the left side first.

CHAKRAS 4, 5

HOTTIE BODY
- sexy shoulders
- relaxed neck
- radiant face
- open chest

IN THE BEDROOM
- Bathing Beauties
- Orgasmic Camel
- Satisfying Side
- Talking in Tongues

hot tip { Do this several times every workday to keep the kinks out of your neck so you're nice and loose when you get home and want to seduce your sweetie.

OPEN WIDE (Sexy Secretary Version) *An instant jaw, neck, and shoulder tension dissolver, this pose is especially good for those who sit for prolonged periods and have a tendency to clench their jaw. You'll be ready for some long, deep kisses after this one.*

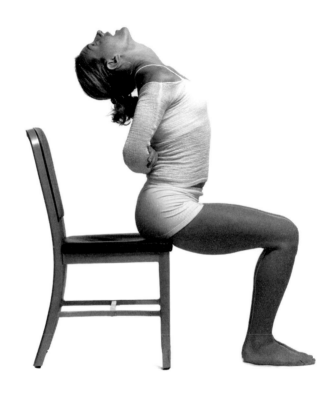

TO DO IT Sit at the edge of a chair with your arms crossed behind your back (near your lower back). Lift your head backward, squeeze your shoulder blades together, and open your chest. Allow your mouth to open naturally. Arch your back.

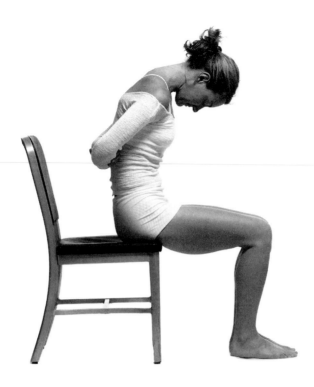

Then drop your head forward, pulling your chin to your chest, and close your mouth. Repeat eight times.

CHAKRAS 2, 4

HOTTIE BODY
- soft neck and throat muscles
- healthy jaw and teeth
- relaxed shoulders

IN THE BEDROOM
- Orgasmic Camel
- Talking in Tongues
- Yin Yang

hot tip **{** Try to keep your jaw relaxed during all of your poses. This is a way to trick your brain into relaxation and enjoyment during exercise—and sex!

SEX KITTEN (Sexy Secretary Version)

This aptly named pose opens the pelvis and lengthens and strengthens the abs and back. This move is a total turn-on for those doing it—and those watching too! Be careful when you do this pose at the office.

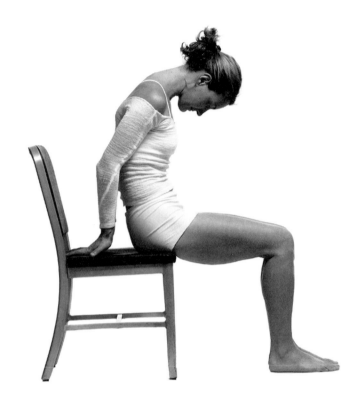

TO DO IT Seated at the edge of your desk chair, place your hands at the back of your chair and bring your back into perfect posture with your head looking downward.

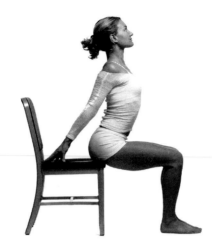

Inhale and arch your back and look slightly upward. Exhale, tuck your tail-bone under, and look at your belly button. Repeat eight times.

CHAKRAS 1 to 7

HOTTIE BODY
· yoga butt
· yummy tummy
· supple back
· relaxed neck
· open heart

IN THE BEDROOM
· Doggie Style
· Double Triangle
· Erotic Froggie
· Orgasmic Camel

hot tip { This pose aids the naturally occurring, but often stagnated, flow of energy needed for sexual drive and explosive orgasms. This flow runs up the front of the torso, through the roof of your mouth, and down the back to the perineum. After you master this pose, you'll definitely feel the difference.

SEXY SHOULDERS (Sexy Secretary Version) *This pose will keep arm and shoulder pain (caused by prolonged mouse use and typing) at bay.*

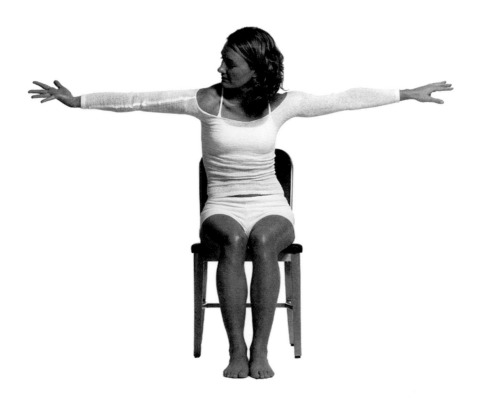

TO DO IT Begin seated at the front of your chair in perfect posture. Place your feet flat on the floor, and raise both arms to shoulder height, parallel to the floor. Rotate your right arm and shoulder forward, and look at your right palm. Repeat four times; then repeat on the other side. Be sure to engage your abdomen and bend forward a little at the waist with each roll.

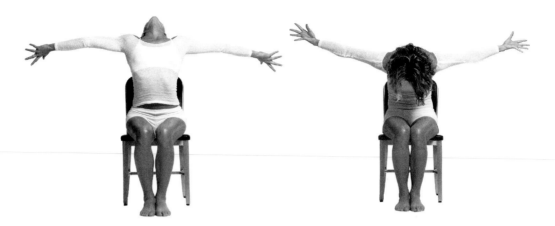

Next inhale and arch your back, looking up at the ceiling and rolling both shoulders backward. Exhale and roll both shoulders forward, making your abdomen hollow, and look at your belly button. Repeat five times, remembering to inhale and exhale fully.

CHAKRAS 2, 4, 5

HOTTIE BODY
· sexy shoulders
· open chest and heart
· perfect posture

IN THE BEDROOM
· The Conquest
· Surf's Up
· Wild Child

hot tip { Blocked shoulders can lead to a blocked heart. Be sure to do this position often if you tend to have a stiff neck and tight shoulders, which are real dampeners on your love life.

SEATED STIMULATION
By now you may understand the importance of your vitality and sexual energy. Don't let the subtleties of this move fool you—it actually works. So don't sit on it . . . encourage it!

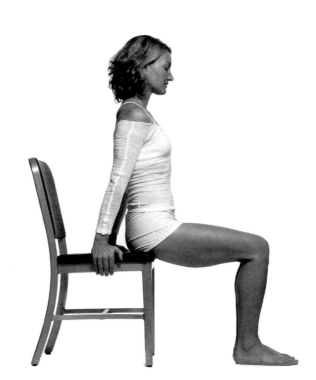

TO DO IT Sitting at the edge of a chair (preferably a hard-bottom chair; or you can place a book under your butt), plant your feet firmly on the floor and sit in correct posture. Using your feet (not your upper body), push back and forth on the floor until you notice your pelvis and sit bones gently rocking forward and back. This is a subtle yet completely effective stimulation for the perineum and genital organs. Rock for about thirty seconds.

**HOTTIE
BODY**
· yummy tummy
· strong obliques

**IN THE
BEDROOM**
· Rearview
· Rock Steady

hot tip {

Be careful, ladies: This one can be quite stimulating to the external genitalia and clitoris. You might want to wait for the end of day to try this. Or if you're feeling naughty at work, try a lunchtime quickie lovemaking session (just not at the office—find a local hotel room or sneak home for an hour).

FLASHDANCE (Sexy Secretary Version) *If you have your eye on the cutie in the next cubicle over, this pose will be a wakeup call for him. Oh, if only there were a bucket of water suspended over your desk! Remember Jennifer Beals in the film* Flashdance?

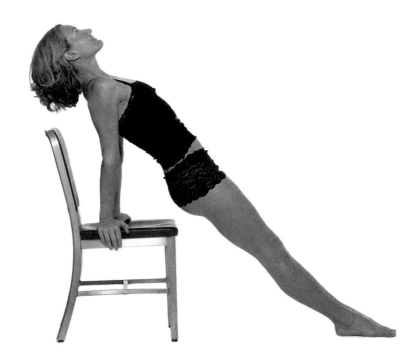

TO DO IT Firmly grasp the sides of your chair. Lift your bottom off the chair and extend your legs forward until they are straight, making a plank-like pose. Keep your knees straight and pointing forward, and squeeze your butt. Your feet should be flat on the floor with your toes pointed forward.

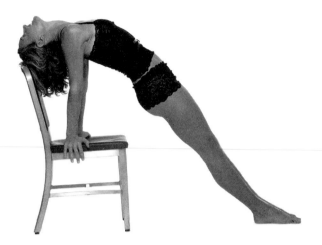

Exhale and tilt your head back to gaze at the ceiling. Then arch your back and point your chest toward the ceiling. Hold for five breaths.

CHAKRAS 2, 3, 4, 5

HOTTIE BODY
- killer inner thighs
- yummy tummy
- yoga butt
- tight triceps

IN THE BEDROOM
- Bridging the Gap
- The Conquest
- Splitting Bamboo

hot tip { If your coworkers get a glimpse of you while doing this, you'll have to beat them off with a stick. Accentuating your breast and throat is always a turn-on.

SEXY SPINAL TWIST (Sexy Secretary Version)

This is another great way to keep your back, abdomen, and all of your internal organs happy. This pose will unkink your back while perfecting your posture.

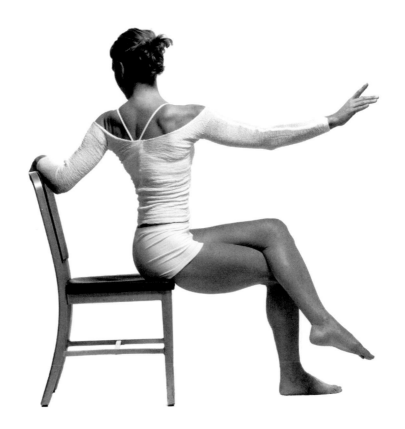

TO DO IT Seated on the edge of your chair, cross your left leg over the right. Place your right hand on your left knee or the edge of your desk and your left hand on the back of the chair.

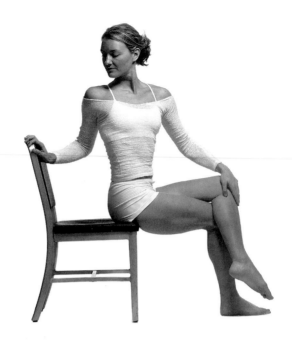

Twist to the right and look over your right shoulder. Take one deep breath into your sexual core. Then uncross and cross your legs in the opposite direction and repeat on the other side. Repeat five times on each side.

CHAKRAS 2, 3, 4

HOTTIE BODY
- whittled waist
- yoga butt
- sexy shoulders

IN THE BEDROOM
- Backseat Buddies
- Rearview
- Satisfying Side

hot tip { Use your shoulders to facilitate a deeper twist in your torso. This will keep your back unkinked for those sexual moments that really matter.

HULA HIPS (Sexy Secretary Version) *A fun and groovy pose, this move adds a little "swerve" into your workday while improving pelvic flexibility. When practiced regularly, Hula Hips can prevent sacral fusion (fusion of the sacrum to the hip bones), a common condition of inactive office workers.*

TO DO IT

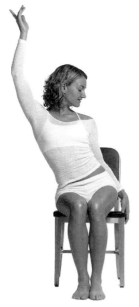

Sit at the front of your chair in perfect posture. Put your hands on the sides of your waist, thumbs in front and fingers in the back, and swivel your torso clockwise, moving at approximately three seconds per circuit. Once you get the hang of it, move your hands chest high, like a hula dancer, and then be creative—try holding them above your head.

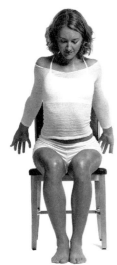

As you move your hips forward, inhale and contract your PC muscles.

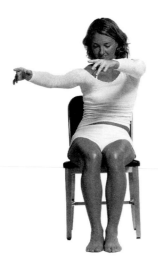

As you move backward, exhale and release your PC muscles. Arch your back and push your chest forward, move your hips to one side curving your waistline, then tuck your tailbone under and around your back. Move in smooth, continuous circles ten times, then reverse and move counterclockwise ten times.

CHAKRAS 1, 2, 3

HOTTIE BODY
- whittled waist
- sexy shoulders
- supple back

IN THE BEDROOM
- Oops, I Dropped the Soap!
- Satisfying Side
- Wild Child

hot tip { Keep your feet flat on the floor and feel sexy. Pelvic flexibility is key to great sex, and this pose will help you achieve it. Want to have a lunchtime quickie? Try this hip opener first, then straddle your partner in his chair. Your loose hips will create an unbelievable lap dance.

SECRET BUTT SQUEEZES

This pose is the ultimate secret weapon for better sex because it can be done so discreetly that no one will even know you are doing it. It's a great pose for sculpting the perfect yoga butt. Practice this as often as you can—especially while at your desk, seated while traveling, or while watching TV.

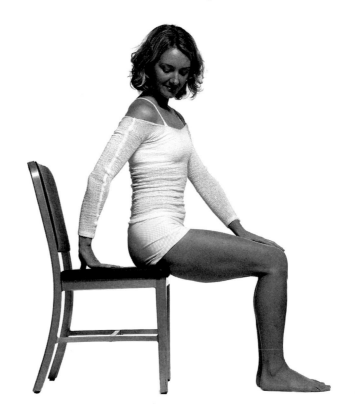

TO DO IT Sit in a desk chair, and keep both feet planted on the floor. Contract your glutes (think of the crease where your leg meets your butt). This is a just a little squeeze, isolating the small yet important area of your gluteus, which firms and lifts your butt. First, contract only the right side of your butt thirty-two times, then repeat on the left side thirty-two times. Then squeeze both sides together twenty-four times. Oooooh, it hurts so good!

CHAKRAS 1, 2

HOTTIE BODY
- yoga butt
- perfect posture
- glorious glutes

IN THE BEDROOM
- Doggie Style
- Double Triangle
- Erotic Froggie
- Oops, I Dropped the Soap!
- Rearview

hot tip { You'll know that you are doing this correctly when your butt wiggles and lifts up on the side you are squeezing. Your partner will notice a difference, so wake up and start squeezing.

SEATED FORWARD BEND (Sexy Secretary Version)

This pose tones the leg muscles while stretching out the hamstrings, neck, and back. It also allows for a rush of blood and energy to flood the brain, which provides a fresh perspective, increased vigor, and enhanced facial beauty.

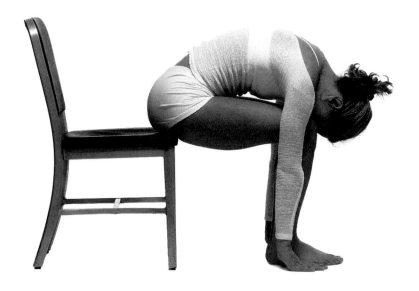

TO DO IT Sit in perfect posture at the front of a chair. Let your arms be at your sides, in line with your shoulders. Lower your chin to your chest, and roll all the way forward, touching your hands to the floor. Hold, relax, and take five deep breaths.

CHAKRAS 1, 2, 5

HOTTIE BODY
- relaxed neck
- yummy tummy
- flexible lower back
- radiant face

IN THE BEDROOM
- Backward-Forward Bend
- Bathing Beauties
- Bundled Package
- Splitting Bamboo

hot tip { Remember to breathe deeply into your sexual core and let the energy flow.

KILLER HIP OPENER (Sexy Secretary Version)

This pose stretches the hips and sends a rush of blood to your muscles there. It can be a bit painful at first, but if you are gentle and consistent, you'll achieve killer results.

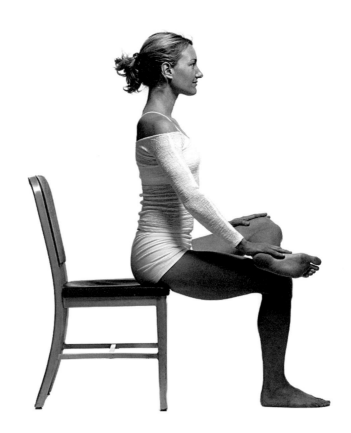

TO DO IT While seated in your desk chair, bend your left knee and cross the ankle over your right thigh. Place one hand on your knee and the other on your ankle. Keep your right foot flat on the floor and hold your back tall.

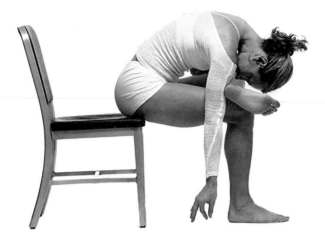

Exhale and bend at the waist, keeping your chin lifted at first, and then dropping the chin to touch your shin. Hold for three breaths.

CHAKRAS 2, 3

HOTTIE BODY
· loose hips
· pliable pelvis
· relaxed neck

IN THE BEDROOM
· Backseat Buddies
· Erotic Froggie
· Rock Steady

hot tip { Keep your abdomen contracted to protect your lower back from pinching. Also make sure to keep your neck relaxed. Open hips keep your sexual energy flowing all day long. You never know when a surprise quickie might happen.

5

CORE ROUTINES

Welcome to the core routines. By now you've sampled some of our hot and sexy poses and maybe even sampled some of our even hotter sex positions at the end of the book. We know you've already taken a sneak peek. Now it's time to focus that sexual energy. Try one core routine three times a week and slowly build up to thirty to forty-five minutes of practice. There's even one routine—Macho Man (page 226)—for you to try with the hottie in your life. Don't worry, he'll thank you later, after a few sessions of this routine, when he realizes his staying power is greatly extended.

The Honeymoon

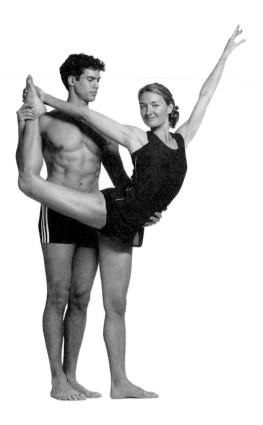

Be inventive, spicy, and bountiful in your lovemaking

The honeymoon should never end! Whether you're going on your third, fifth, or fifteenth anniversary—or you're about to get married—this routine will put you in the best physical and sexual shape ever. The Honeymoon is our most challenging routine of all and will definitely yield top results. A healthy and active sex life is one of the most important keys to a happy marriage or relationship. It is also one of the first things we shelve when our lives get too busy. Make time for a hot sex life, and get in shape for it too. Remember what it was like when you first met, how you couldn't keep your hands off each other? Wouldn't you like to get that feeling back? You can! The

Honeymoon works out the sexual core with moves like Candy Cane, Camel, and Hello, while encouraging you to breathe life into your sex organs and sexual energy centers. As a result, sex positions such as Orgasmic Camel, Double Triangle, and Yin Yang will be a breeze. Practicing this core routine, which addresses all of your chakras, can help to increase honor, respect, and love. Just reading about this routine will get you warm and fuzzy all over!

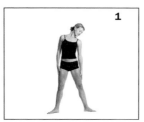

1. Neck and Shoulder Release (page 160)

2. **BASIC BEAUTY** (page 42)

3. **SUN SALUTATION** (page 38)

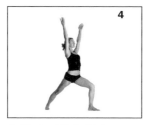

4. Warrior I (left side) (page 134)

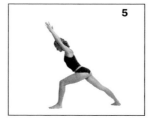

5. Crave (left side) (page 136)

6. Repeat #4 and 5 on the other side.

7. **SUN SALUTATION** (page 38)

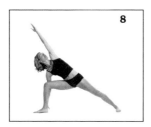

8. Side Angle (each side) (page 156)

9. **SUN SALUTATION** (page 38)

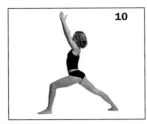

10. Warrior I—Crescent Variation (left side) (page 135)

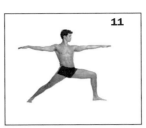

11. Warrior II (left side) (page 138)

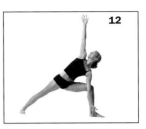

12. Bent-Knee Triangle (left side) (page 152)

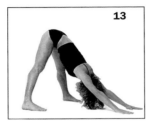

13. Open Wide (left side) (page 140)

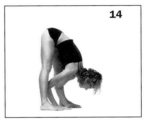

14. Open Wide—Variation (left side) (page 141)

15. Repeat #10 to 14 on the other side.

16. **SUN SALUTATION** (page 38)

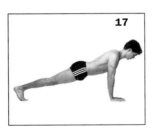

17. Plank (page 44)

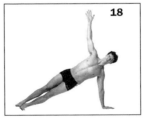

18. Plank Pose Side (each side) (page 46)

19. **SUN SALUTATION** (page 38)

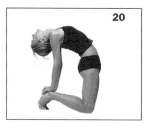

20. Camel
(page 62)

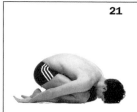

21. Chill Out (page 60)

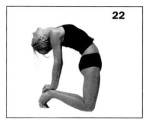

22. Camel
(page 62)

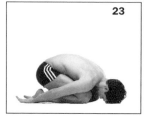

23. Chill Out (page 60)

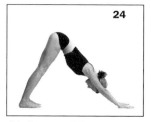

24. Downward Dog (page 130)

25. **SUN SALUTATION** (page 38)

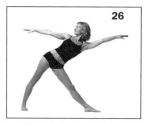

26. Triangle (left side)
(page 150)

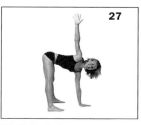

27. Hello (left side)
(page 142)

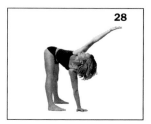

28. Loose Hello (left
side) (page 143)

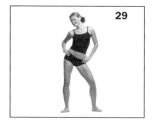

29. Hula Hips (8 times each
side) (page 148)

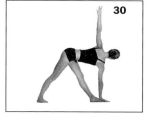

30. Reverse Triangle (left side)
(page 154)

31. Repeat #26 to 30 on the other side.

32. **SUN SALUTATION** (page 38)

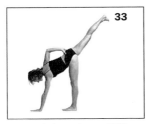

33. Half Moon (page 158)

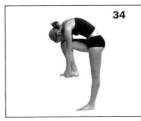

34. Candy Cane (each side) (page 168)

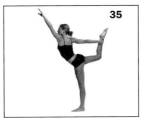

35. Standing Beau (each side) (page 170)

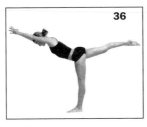

36. Cupid's Arrow (each side) (page 172)

37. *Advanced option:* Repeat Candy Cane, Standing Beau, and Cupid's Arrow on each leg without coming off your standing leg between poses.

38. **SUN SALUTATION** (page 38)

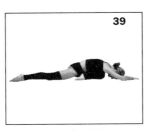

39. Pigeon (left side) (page 70)

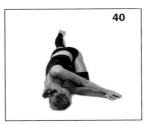

40. Sleeping Pigeon (left side) (page 72)

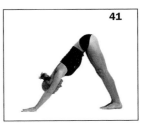

41. Downward Dog (page 130)

42. Repeat #39 to 41 on the other side.

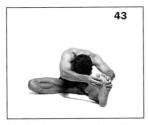

43. Seated Forehead to Knee (left side) (page 112)

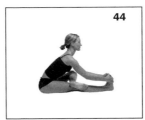

44. Killer Hip Opener (left side) (page 104)

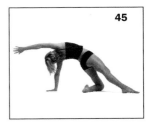

45. Half Back Bend (page 114)

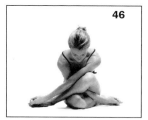

46

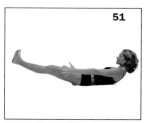

47

46. Almost Lotus (page 116)   47. Boat (page 118)

48. Repeat #43 to 47 on the other side.

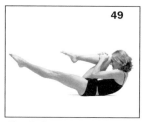

49

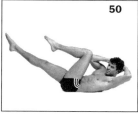

50

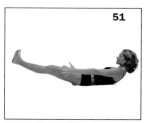

51

49. Ab Switches (8 times)
   (page 76)

50. Yogacycles (8 slow,
   16 fast, 8 slow, 16 fast)
   (page 74)

51. Ballet Belly (4 times)
   (page 78)

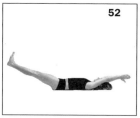

52

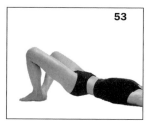

53

52. Karate Body (8 times)
   (page 80)

53. Pelvic Squeezes
   (16 each position) (page 84)

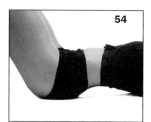

54

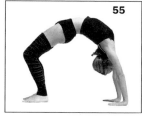

55

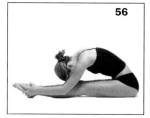

56

54. Bump Bump Bump
   (8 times) (page 86)

55. Bridge (page 92)

56. Seated Forward
   Bend (page 94)

57. Breath of Fire (30 breaths first set, 60 breaths second set) (page 24)

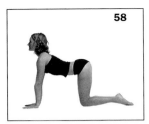

58. Sex Kitten (8 times) (page 52)

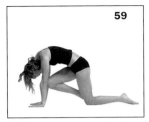

59. Sex Kitten (variation) (8 times each side) (page 53)

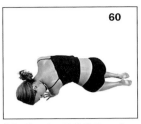

60. Chasing Tail (8 times) (page 54)

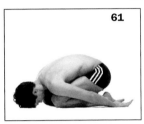

61. Chill Out (page 60)

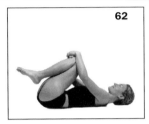

62. Wind-Relieving (page 120)

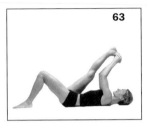

63. Of Great Benefit (right side) (page 122)

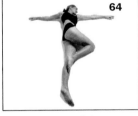

64. Easy Spinal Twist (page 124)

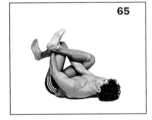

65. Rear Release (page 126)

66. Repeat #62 to 65 on the other side.

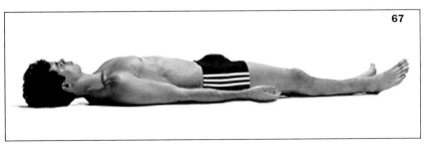

67. At Peace (full 5 minutes) (page 128)

Hot Date Prep

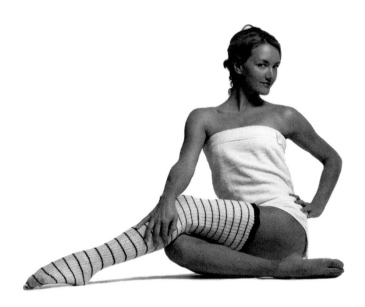

This predate yoga blast gets you in shape and turned on fast

Who has time to drive to the gym and back? In the convenience of your own living room, this routine covers all your important assets and gets you date ready—and quick! This challenging core routine firms your rear, tones your shoulders and arms, flattens your belly, and gets you relaxed and glowing before you head out. Tweaking chakras 1, 2, 3, and 5, you'll be calm, cool, and collected when you step out on the town. The attention to deep breathing in Hot Date Prep will develop your sexual core and keep any predate jitters at bay. So remember, before you dress, release stress—and get ready to turn heads!

1. **BASIC BEAUTY** (page 42)

2. **SUN SALUTATION** (page 38)

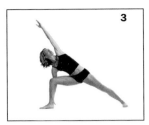

3. Side Angle (each side) (page 156)

4. SUN SALUTATION (page 38)

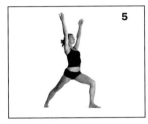 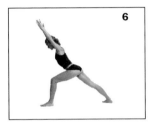

5. Warrior I (left side) (page 134)

6. Crave (left side) (page 136)

7. Repeat #5 and 6 on the other side.

8. SUN SALUTATION (page 38)

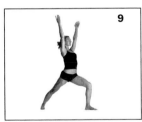 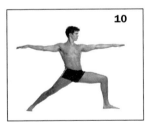 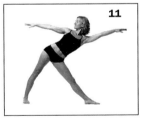

9. Warrior I (left side) (page 134)

10. Warrior II (left side) (page 138)

11. Triangle (left side) (page 150)

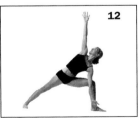 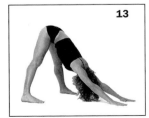

12. Bent-Knee Triangle (left side) (page 152)

13. Open Wide (left side) (page 140)

14. Repeat #9 to 13 on the other side.

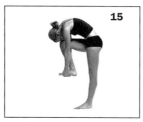

15. Candy Cane (each side) (page 168)

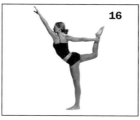

16. Standing Beau (each side) (page 170)

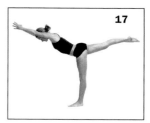

17. Cupid's Arrow (each side) (page 172)

18. *Advanced option:* Repeat Candy Cane, Standing Beau, and Cupid's Arrow on each leg without coming off the standing leg between poses.

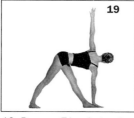

19. Reverse Triangle (each side) (page 154)

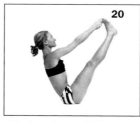

20. Boat (page 118)

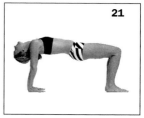

21. Tabletop (page 100)

22. Repeat #20 to 21 four times.

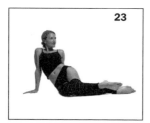

23. Sexy Spinal Twist (4 times) (page 110)

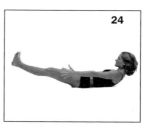

24. Ballet Belly (8 times) (page 78)

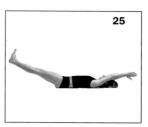

25. Karate Body (8 times) (page 80)

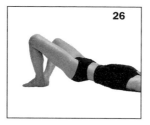

26. Pelvic Squeezes (8 times each position) (page 84)

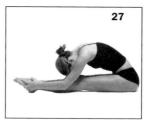

27. Seated Forward Bend (page 94)

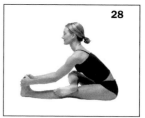

28. Killer Hip Opener (each side) (page 104)

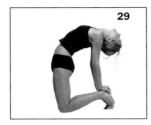

29. Camel (page 62)

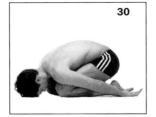

30. Chill Out (page 60)

31. Repeat #29 to 30 two times.

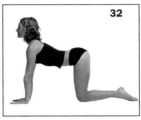

32. Sex Kitten (page 52)

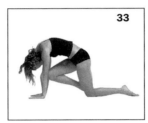

33. Sex Kitten—Variation
(4 times each side)
(page 53)

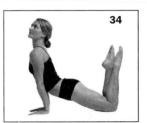

34. Mermaid (page 64)

35. Breath of Fire (30 breaths first set, 60 breaths second set) (page 24)

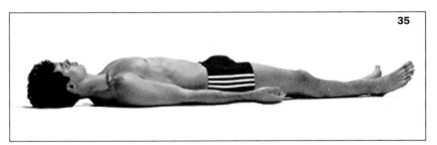

36. At Peace (10 minutes with a hot or cold pack on face) (page 128)

Macho Man

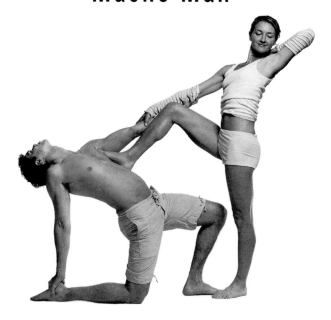

Sweep her off her feet . . . literally

This routine is amped with a bit more yang energy for the man in your life—but you can give it a try too. It taps into the masculine, earthy, strong, and powerful side—the side men are trying to build. Remind him that powerful muscles, a looser lower back, and manly virility will surely be noticed after only a few weeks. Yoga creates long, lean, and beautifully sculpted muscles that your man's regular gym workout just can't achieve. We suggest your partner practice this core session at least twice a week and enhance it by practicing the Dynamic Duo (page 233) for your Saturday morning loving. Tell him that chicks dig it when men think to include them in their fitness and fun, especially if there may be a good roll in the hay afterward. Really! In addition, we've included techniques that, when practiced during sex, help to extend both of your pleasure during the arousal state. This makes sharing your sexual satisfaction in sync with your sweetie more probable. Imagine your man in the Plank and you in Bump Bump Bump; with combined breathing and sexual core strength, you can be in charge of when you will peak.

1. **BASIC BEAUTY** (page 42)

2. **SUN SALUTATION** (page 38)

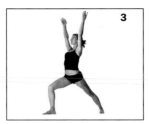

3. Warrior I (each side) (page 134)

4. **SUN SALUTATION** (page 38)

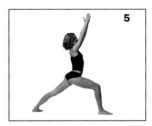

5. Warrior I—Palms Together Variation (each side) (page 134)

6. **SUN SALUTATION** (page 38)

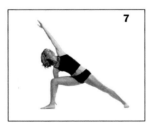

7. Side Angle (each side) (page 156)

8. **SUN SALUTATION** (page 38)

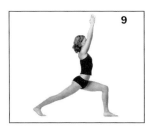

9. Warrior I—Crescent Variation (left side) (page 135)

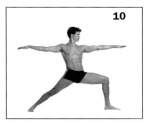

10. Warrior II (left side) (page 138)

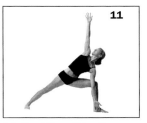

11. Bent-Knee Triangle (left side) (page 152)

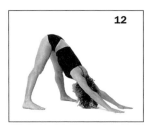

12. Open Wide (left side) (page 140)

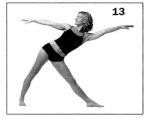

13. Triangle (left side) (page 150)

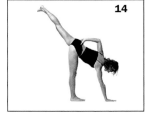

14. Half Moon (left side) (page 158)

15. Repeat #9 to 14 on the other side.

16. **SUN SALUTATION** (page 38)

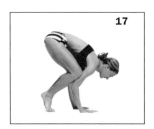

17. Crane (page 58)

18. Repeat #16 to 17 two times.

19. **SUN SALUTATION** (page 38)

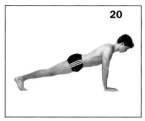
20. Plank (page 44)

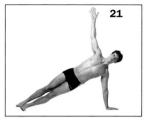
21. Plank Pose Side (each side) (page 46)

22. SUN SALUTATION (page 38)

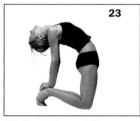
23. Camel (page 62)

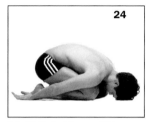
24. Chill Out (page 60)

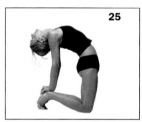
25. Camel (page 62)

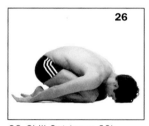
26. Chill Out (page 60)

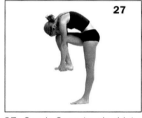
27. Candy Cane (each side) (page 168)

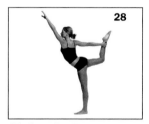
28. Standing Beau (each side) (page 170)

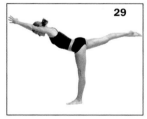
29. Cupid's Arrow (each side) (page 172)

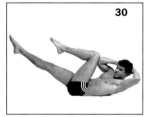
30. Yogacycles (40 times) (page 74)

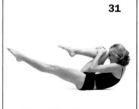
31. Ab Switches (8 times) (page 76)

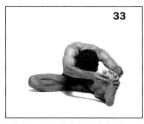

32. Ballet Belly (8 times)
(page 78)

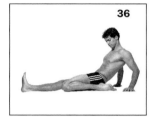

33. Seated Forehead to Knee
(each side) (page 112)

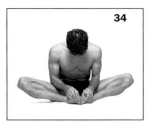

34. Butterfly (page 108)

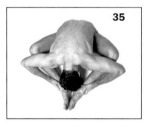

35. Extended Butterfly
(page 109)

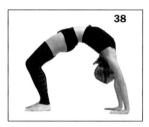

36. Diamond (each side)
(page 106)

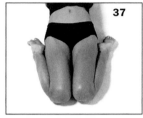

37. Full Diamond
(page 107)

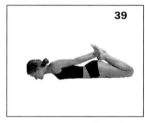

38. Bridge (page 92)

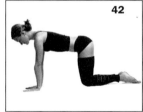

39. Floor Bow (page 68)

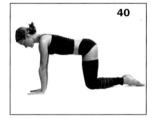

40. On All Fours (page 50)

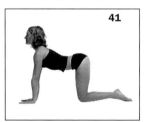

41. Sex Kitten (page 52)

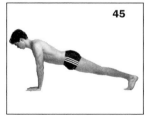

42. On All Fours (page 50)

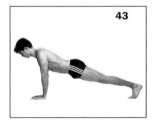

43. Plank (page 44)

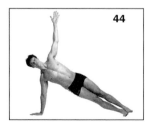

44. Plank Pose Side
(page 46)

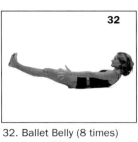

45. Plank (page 44)

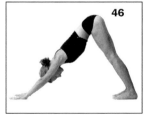

46. Downward Dog
(page 130)

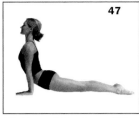
47. Upward Dog (page 48)

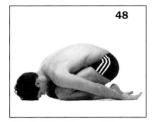
48. Chill Out (page 60)

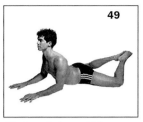
49. Froggie (page 56)

50. Breath of Fire (30 breaths first set, 60 breaths second set) (page 24)

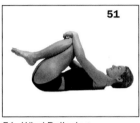
51. Wind-Relieving
(page 120)

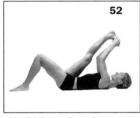
52. Of Great Benefit
(page 122)

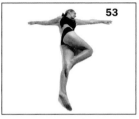
53. Easy Spinal Twist
(page 124)

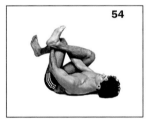
54. Rear Release (page 126)

55. Repeat #51 to 54 on the other side.

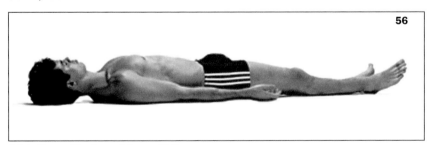
56. At Peace (5 minutes) (page 128)

6

QUICKIE ROUTINES

Whether you're single and dating like Samantha or settled with a kid like Miranda, these targeted routines will keep you coming back for more. And believe us, your partner won't be complaining either. Add these quickie routines to your core ones when you're looking for a little extra oomph in your sex life. The Peep Show is one of our favorites and will surely add some spice to your romance as you tease your sweetie with some naughty poses. Fantasy and creativity in sex are great ways to add variety and put to use all of the bending, twisting, and squeezing techniques you've learned. These may be quick routines but, trust us, the sex will be long-lasting.

Dynamic Duo

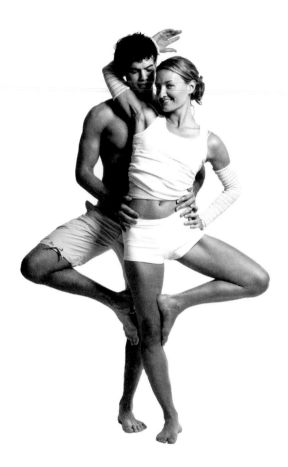

For daring and caring couples

The dynamic duo is the ultimate in foreplay! It's the perfect way to shake off daily tension and move into a loving and sensual state of mind before bedtime, or even as a Saturday morning rise-and-shine! You don't even have to change out of your PJs. For a total turn-on, synchronize your breathing, move together, and fall into an easy and natural rhythm together. Giving a helpful adjustment in a pose is a sensuous way to spend time . . . and who knows where it can lead? So stretch, open, and awaken all of your body parts and get ready to sweat a little—or a lot.

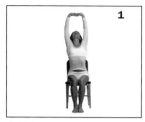

1. Upholding Heaven (4 times) (page 190)

2. **SUN SALUTATION** (page 38)

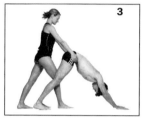

3. Duo Downward Dog
   (page 176)

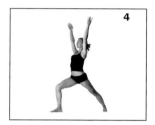

4. Warrior I (each side) (page 134)

5. **SUN SALUTATION** (page 38)

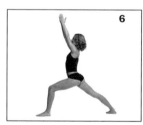

6. Warrior I—Palms Together
   Variation (left side) (page 134)

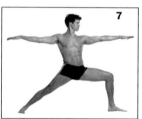

7. Warrior II (left side)
   (page 138)

8. **SUN SALUTATION** (page 38)

9. Repeat #6 to 8 on the other side.

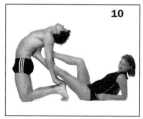

10. Duo Camel (page 186)

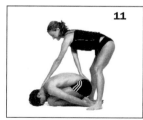

11. Duo Chill Out with
    Massage (page 188)

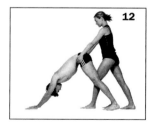

12. Duo Downward Dog
    (page 176)

13. **SUN SALUTATION** (page 38)

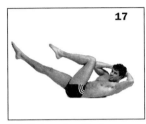
14. Open Wide (page 140)

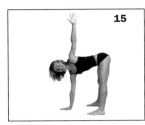
15. Hello (page 142)

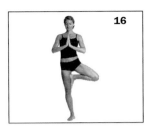
16. Tree (each side) (page 174)

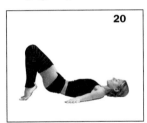
17. Yogacycles (8 slow, 8 fast, then repeat) (page 74)

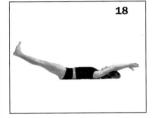
18. Karate Body (8 times) (page 80)

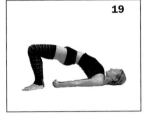
19. Half Bridge (page 90)

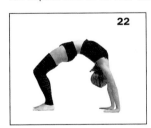
20. Belly Roll (page 88)

21. Repeat #19 to 20 four times slowly.

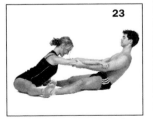
22. Bridge (page 92)

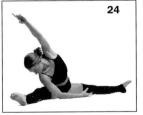
23. Dunking for Apples (facing each other) (page 182)

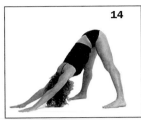
24. Sidesaddle (each side) (page 98)

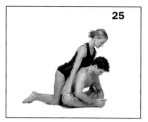

25. Duo Butterfly (page 180)   26. Duo Extended Butterfly (page 181)

27. Breath of Fire (30 breaths first set, 60 breaths second set) (page 24)

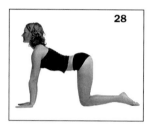

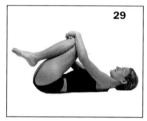

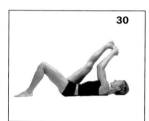

28. Sex Kitten (page 52)

29. Wind-Relieving (page 120)

30. Of Great Benefit (page 122)

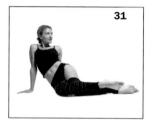

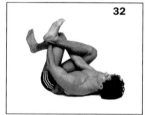

31. Sexy Spinal Twist (page 110)

32. Rear Release (page 126)

33. Repeat #29 to 32 on the other side.

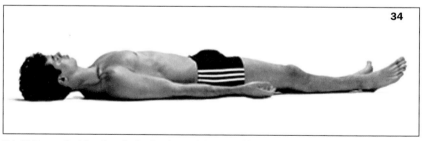

34. At Peace (holding hands for 8 minutes) (page 128)

Bedtime Bootie

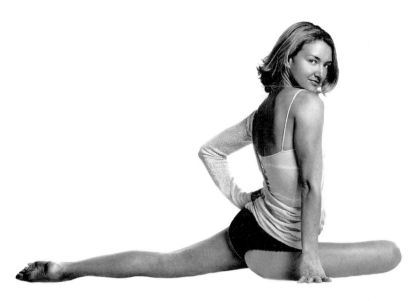

A quick firm and tone for a bodacious bootie before bedtime action

This quick and fabulous routine is designed to work anywhere, and you can do it any time you want to rev up your body before hitting the sheets. Do it together or on your own. This quick yoga blast will firm up your rear and lower back in just fifteen minutes and is great if you tend to sit a lot during the day. Driving, flying, and just sitting at a desk can make for a flat, deflated, sore, or weak derriere. Bedtime Bootie with Locust and Pelvic Squeezes is the perfect solution! Bring new appeal to your backside by practicing the supplemental Bedtime Bootie routine twice a week (or more if you've had a long day of traveling or sitting). One final note: Trapped wind in the intestines can make for uncomfortable, embarrassing, and downright unbearable sex. That's why we've included Wind-Relieving in this routine.

1. Breath of Fire (30 breaths first set, 60 breaths second set) (page 24)

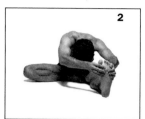

2. Seated Forehead to Knee (left side) (page 112)

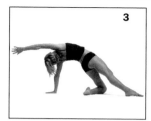

3. Half Back Bend (page 114)

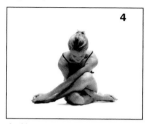

4. Almost Lotus (page 116)

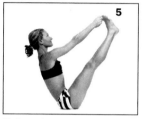

5. Boat (page 118)

6. Repeat #2 to 5 on the other side.

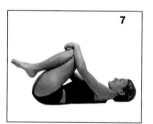

7. Wind-Relieving (page 120)

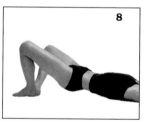

8. Pelvic Squeezes (16 times each position) (page 84)

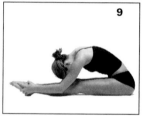

9. Seated Forward Bend (page 94)

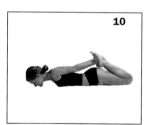

10. Floor Bow (2 times) (page 68)

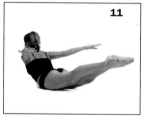

11. Locust (2 times) (page 66)

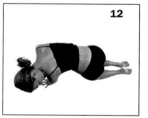

12. Chasing Tail (8 times each side) (page 54)

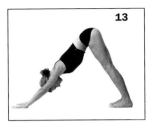

13. Downward Dog (page 130)

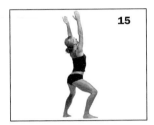

14. Half Moon (page 158)

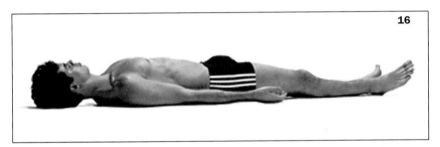

15. Modern Breath (8 times) (page 144)

16. At Peace (2 minutes) (page 128)

Sexy Secretary

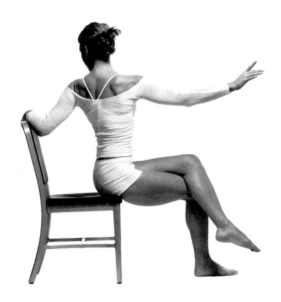

Your little at-work secret can be done as often as possible

Does it feel like your boss is riding you a little too hard lately? (No, not that way!) Do you find that your body has taken on an uncanny resemblance to your desk chair? Sounds like you need the Sexy Secretary to come to your rescue. This routine releases office neck and shoulders (chronic pain caused by excessive computer and desk work), and lower back tightness. It also tones the abs, butt, and arms—all while you are sitting at your desk. Keeping your spine active and supple will balance all of your chakras, particularly the first and second, which are most damaged by inactivity, negativity, and sitting. When done on a regular basis, this routine will prevent repetitive strain injuries and reduce emotional stress and strain. Most important, it will get your focus back where it belongs: on your sex life! Lowered libido, weak and sore lower back, sexual dysfunction, stiffness (and not where it counts), uptight back neck and shoulders, and depression are just a few of the symptoms linked to prolonged periods of sitting. Hunched over a computer—this is not sexy. But we have just the thing to perk you up!

We love the Seated Stimulation and Secret Butt Squeezes for their libido-boosting power—and no one ever has to know that you're doing them! Since you have to work to earn money to pay for your fabulous lifestyle, at least you can use your on-the-job time to beef up your sexual energy.

Say no to the three o'clock candy bar or triple espresso with whipped cream and practice the Sexy Secretary instead. Do this at least once a day (but more is definitely better), and find that the daily grind may put a little bump in your nightlife.

Note: All of these poses are the versions found in the Sexy Secretary section of the book.

1. Breath of Fire (30 breaths first set, 60 breaths second set) (page 24)

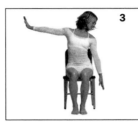

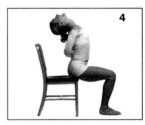

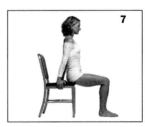

2. Upholding Heaven (4 times) (page 190)

3. Neck and Shoulder Release (page 192)

4. Open Wide (page 194)

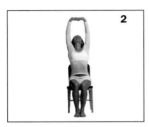

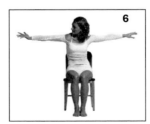

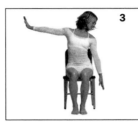

5. Sex Kitten (page 196)

6. Sexy Shoulders (page 198)

7. Seated Stimulation (page 200)

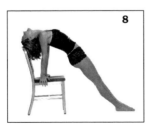

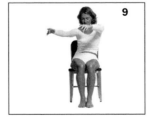

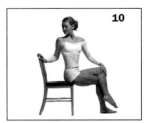

8. Flashdance (2 times) (page 202)

9. Hula Hips (page 206)

10. Sexy Spinal Twist (4 times) (page 204)

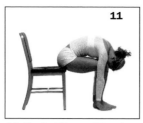

11. Seated Forward Bend
(page 210)

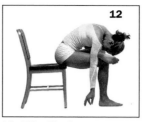

12. Killer Hip Opener
(page 212)

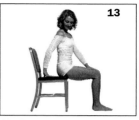

13. Secret Butt Squeezes
(16 times) (page 208)

Peep Show

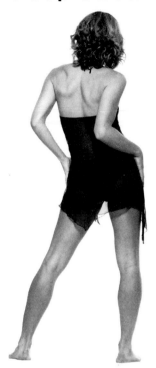

(Hardly) Subtle Seduction

Designed especially for those of you who like to put on that itty-bitty nightie you've been stashing in your top drawer. After all, having an audience makes working out way more erotic. And being in command and showing him what you want will keep your fifth chakra happy and your lines of communication open. Flirty and downright daring for yoga, the steamy and sexy Peep Show will get both of your hearts racing, even though only one of you is actually moving.

He'll be amazed at how flexible you truly are! These moves will prime not only your sexual core, but his as well. The idea is for you and your honey to both get so hot that you never, in fact, complete this routine. Do we really need to tell you how often to do this one? As often as possible, of course! So let go of all inhibitions, dim the lights, and get ready for action. Voyeurism can be such fun.

1. **BASIC BEAUTY** (page 42)

2. **SUN SALUTATION** (page 38)

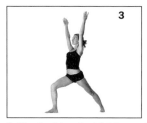

3. Warrior I (each side) (page 134)

4. **SUN SALUTATION** (page 38)

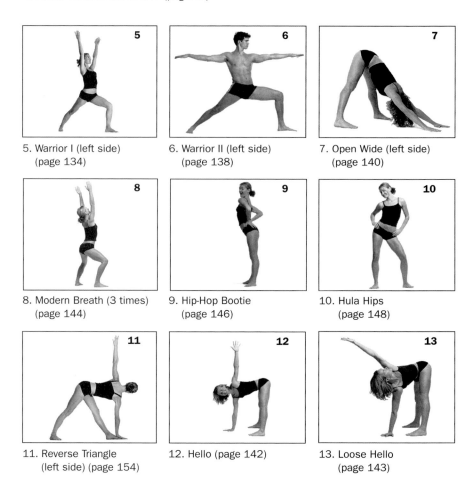

5. Warrior I (left side)
   (page 134)

6. Warrior II (left side)
   (page 138)

7. Open Wide (left side)
   (page 140)

8. Modern Breath (3 times)
   (page 144)

9. Hip-Hop Bootie
   (page 146)

10. Hula Hips
    (page 148)

11. Reverse Triangle
    (left side) (page 154)

12. Hello (page 142)

13. Loose Hello
    (page 143)

14. Repeat #5 to 13 on the other side.

15. Transition to the floor by walking feet and hands together and squat down.

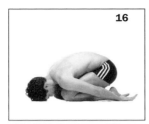

16. Chill Out (page 60)

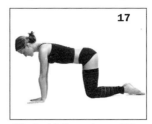

17. On All Fours (page 50)

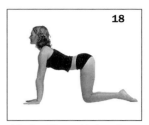

18. Sex Kitten (4 times) (page 52)

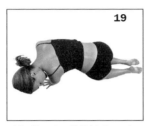

19. Chasing Tail (4 times) (page 54)

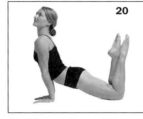

20. Mermaid (page 64)

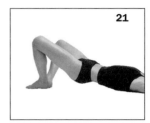

21. Pelvic Squeezes (4 times each position) (page 84)

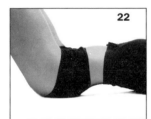

22. Bump Bump Bump (4 times) (page 86)

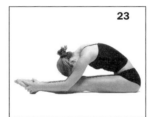

23. Seated Forward Bend (page 94)

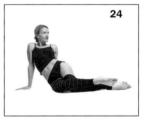

24. Sexy Spinal Twist (4 times) (page 110)

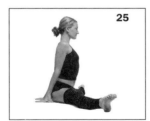

25. In the Saddle (page 96)

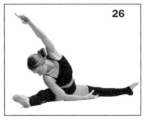

26. Sidesaddle (each side) (page 98)

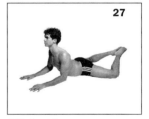

27. Froggie (page 56)

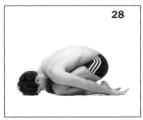

28. Chill Out (4 minutes) (page 60)

Flexy Makes Sexy

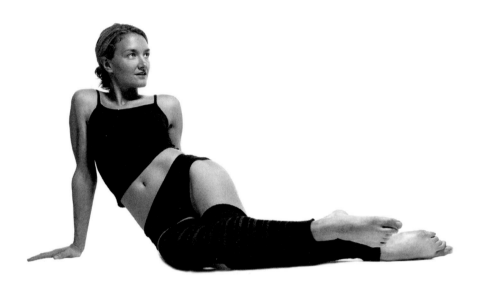

Being bendable has its perks

Do you want to try poses in the bedroom that you've never before dared? Backseat Buddies, Bathing Beauties, and Oops, I Dropped the Soap! should be adequate incentive. Try our Flexy Makes Sexy routine, a quick and powerful weapon that increases the flexibility of both your body and mind. Maintaining a stretchable body prevents strains and pains and also combats boredom in the bedroom. With your newfound flexibility, you may find yourself suggesting wild positions in places you never dreamed possible. Have you thought about that tiny airplane bathroom? Try out this routine for that little extra oomph in your love life.

1. **BASIC BEAUTY** (page 42)

2. **SUN SALUTATION** (page 38)

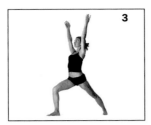

3. Warrior I (page 134)

4. **SUN SALUTATION** (page 38)

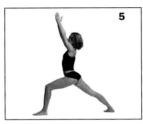

5. Warrior I—Palms Together
Variation (left side)
(page 134)

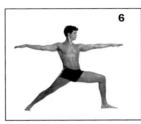

6. Warrior II (left side)
(page 138)

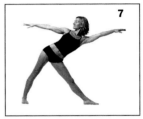

7. Triangle (left side)
(page 150)

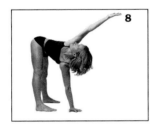

8. Loose Hello (page 143)

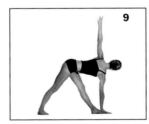

9. Reverse Triangle (left side)
(page 154)

10. Repeat #5 to 9 on the other side.

11. **SUN SALUTATION** (page 38)

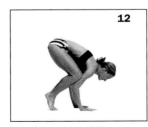

12. Crane (page 58)

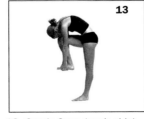

13. Candy Cane (each side)
(page 168)

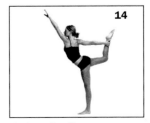

14. Standing Beau
(each side) (page 170)

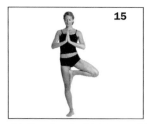

15. Tree (each side) (page 174)

16. **SUN SALUTATION** (page 38)

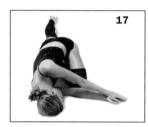

17. Sleeping Pigeon (each side) (page 72)

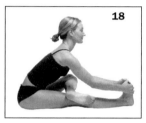

18. Killer Hip Opener (left side) (page 104)

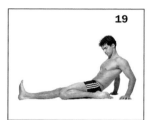

19. Diamond (page 106)

20. Repeat #18 to 19 on the other side.

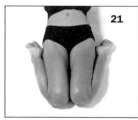

21. Full Diamond (page 106)

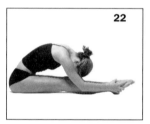

22. Seated Forward Bend (page 94)

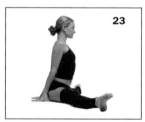

23. In the Saddle (page 96)

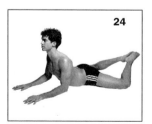

24. Froggie (page 56)

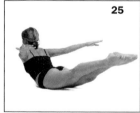

25. Locust (page 66)

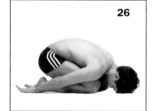

26. Chill Out (page 60)

27. Breath of Fire (30 breaths slower, one set only) (page 24)

Not Tonight, I Have a Headache

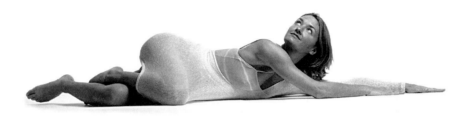

A gentle restorative little nudge

Sometimes stress, fatigue, and a hectic schedule suck the sex drive right out of us. When this happens, try our Not Tonight, I Have a Headache routine, which is a gentle, relaxing, and brief series of poses that targets the pain or exhaustion you may be feeling and gives your body the love it deserves. So close the door, dim the lights, and gently unwind. Couples who are craving closeness and intimacy but are too exhausted to make love can do this quickie routine together. You may find you're in the mood after all, or maybe you just feel calm and rested. Either way, there's nothing like this routine to get you back to feeling relaxed, happy, and centered. Breath deeply and slowly into you sexual core and third chakra for a total energy overhaul.

For some of us, learning to let go into the stillness of At Peace position can be the hardest part of this routine. At Peace pose is an essential aspect of all yoga. It is the only *Better Sex Through Yoga* pose that requires no physical effort, only a willingness to let go. When mastered, At Peace will bring peace of mind, regeneration, and completion to your yoga flows.

1. **BASIC BEAUTY** (page 42)

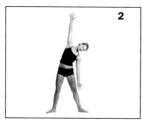

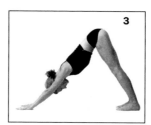

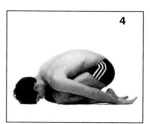

2. Neck and Shoulder Release (page 160)

3. Downward Dog (page 130)

4. Chill Out (page 60)

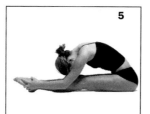

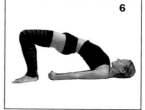

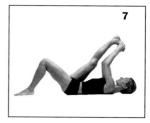

5. Seated Forward Bend (squeeze all toes) (page 94)

6. Half Bridge (page 90)

7. Of Great Benefit (left side) (page 122)

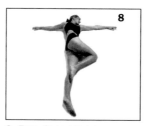

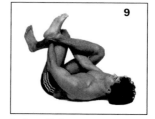

8. Easy Spinal Twist (page 124)

9. Rear Release (page 126)

10. Repeat #7 to 9 on the other side.

11. Three-Part Breath (on back, 8 times) (page 25)

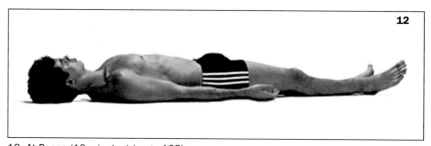

12. At Peace (10 minutes) (page 128)

Between the Sheets

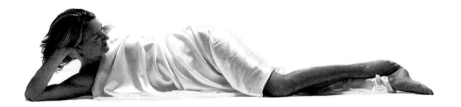

A quickie before a quickie

Maybe you blew off your core routine today, or you just can't get enough of that great loving feeling that comes from a really great *Better Sex Through Yoga* session. Here's a quickie routine that hits some major points of interest in less than five minutes. And it's done in bed! Between the Sheets is our fast, loose, hot, super-stretchy so-you-can-have-sex-routine. This targeted abdomen-firming, hip-opening, back-stretching, and butt-tightening session gets you fresh and ready for a flawless romp with your sweetie. Sex positions like Doggie Style and Splitting Bamboo are just around the corner. It's easy. Wait for your love to step into the bathroom before bed, and run through this routine before he gets back. He won't know what hit him!

1. Breath of Fire (60 quick breaths) (page 24)

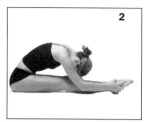

2. Seated Forward Bend (page 94)

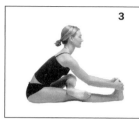

3. Killer Hip Opener (each side) (page 104)

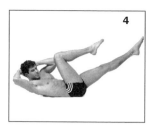

4. Yogacycles (8 slow, 8 quick) (page 74)

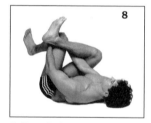

5. Wind-Relieving (page 120)

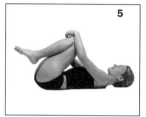

6. Of Great Benefit (page 122)

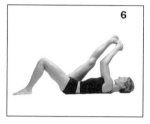

7. Easy Spinal Twist (page 124)

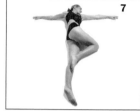

8. Rear Release (page 126)

9. Repeat #5 to 8 on the other side.

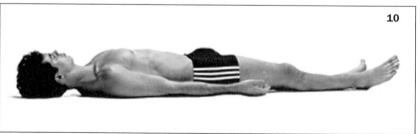

10. At Peace (rest for the few minutes it takes for your lover to appear) (page 128)

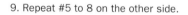

Like a Virgin

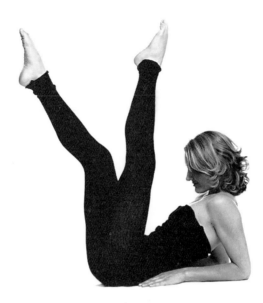

Find your sexual core of prepregnancy yore

Has your sex life been reduced to a quick peck on the cheek as your mate runs out the door for work? Do you actually reject you lover's advances when he sensually rubs you from behind? Have you forgotten what the words *libido, horny, aroused,* and *intimacy* mean? If you answered yes to any of these questions, your sex life and potentially your relationship are in danger of extinction. Get it back, girl!

You're going to be so frisky, ready, willing, and oh-so-able after shaping up with Like a Virgin that you'd better put a babysitter for the kids on the payroll because your sex life is coming back in a *big* way.

Start by doing the Like a Virgin flow at least twice a week, in addition to your three core routines, and feel your sexual prowess return. Reacquaint yourself with your postpregnancy body by giving your sexual core muscles, pelvic muscles, and libido the reawakening you deserve. Make them work for you again and start having fun with new sex positions.

1. **BASIC BEAUTY** (page 42)

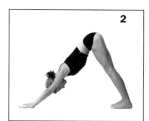

2. Downward Dog
   (hold for 4 breaths)
   (page 130)

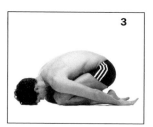

3. Chill Out
   (page 60)

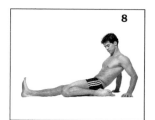

4. Ab Switches
   (16 times) (page 76)

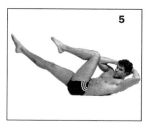

5. Yogacycles (2 sets: 8 slow,
   16 fast, 8 slow)
   (page 74)

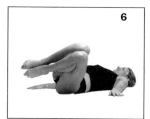

6. Cha Cha Cha
   (4 times) (page 82)

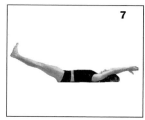

7. Karate Body
   (8 times) (page 80)

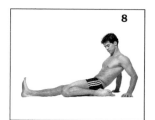

8. Diamond (page 106)

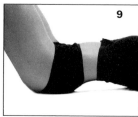

9. Bump Bump Bump
   (16 times each position)
   (page 86)

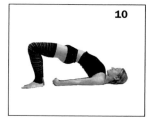

10. Half Bridge
    (page 90)

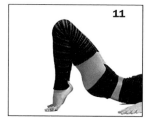

11. Belly Roll (page 88)

12. Repeat #10 to 11 eight times.

13. **SUN SALUTATION** (page 38)

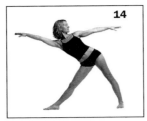

14. Triangle (each side) (page 150)

15. **SUN SALUTATION** (page 38)

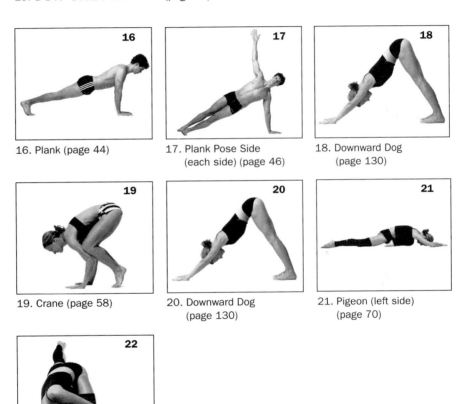

16. Plank (page 44)

17. Plank Pose Side
(each side) (page 46)

18. Downward Dog
(page 130)

19. Crane (page 58)

20. Downward Dog
(page 130)

21. Pigeon (left side)
(page 70)

22. Sleeping Pigeon (left side) (page 72)

23. Repeat #21 to 22 on the other side.

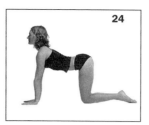

24. Sex Kitten (4 times)
(page 52)

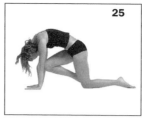

25. Sex Kitten—Variation
(4 times each side)
(page 53)

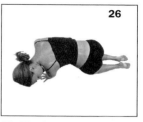

26. Chasing Tail (8 times)
(page 54)

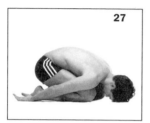

27. Chill Out (page 60)

28. Breath of Fire (30 breaths first set, 60 breaths second set) (page 24)

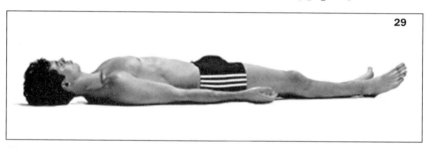

29. At Peace (5 minutes) (page 128)

7

MIND-BLOWING SEX POSITIONS

Admit it, we know you've cheated and skipped ahead to read this chapter already. That's okay. If you haven't, it's well worth the wait. These are all of the sex positions we've been telling you about—the ones that will be so much fun to do and so easy since you've been practicing our *Better Sex Through Yoga* poses.

The absolute *best* reason for boosting your sexual fitness through *Better Sex Through Yoga* is to get into these totally hot sex positions. You may be familiar with some of them. If you're not, don't worry. All of these positions incorporate the *Better Sex Through Yoga* poses explained earlier: Yin Yang, Double Triangle . . . these are seriously killer positions for experiencing better sex.

But don't just take our word for it. Now that you've mastered some of the poses, put them straight into practice. You are going to love the way these creative positions make you feel while making love—they are fun, enticing, and feel good to do. Leave behind your usual bedroom moves for these erotic, playful ones that will bring you closer to your partner and help you have the best sex of your life! Your *Better Sex Through Yoga* sex positions will make it possible for you to fulfill your pleasure goal—whether it's more effective arousal, stronger orgasms, or simply achieving orgasm.

Whatever your sexual goals may be, keep this list of handy positions, and try them *all*. Get inspired, stick to your yoga practice, and soon all of these sex positions will be within easy reach.

BACKSEAT BUDDIES

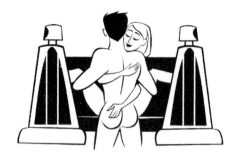

Doing it in the backseat of a car takes some flexibility, but trust us: It's so hot to feel like you're back in high school making out after school. Sit on the backseat with your feet propped up on the back of the front seat. Your partner kneels on the floor in between your legs.

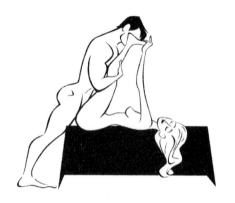

BACKWARD-FORWARD BEND

Lie on your back while your partner stands at the edge of the bed. Both your feet are resting on his shoulders as he penetrates and leans close to you. Your body is bent like a Duo Seated Forward Bend.

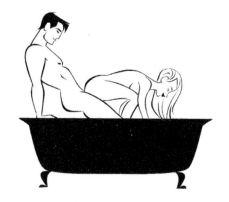

BATHING BEAUTIES

While in the tub, crouch over your partner in the Crane pose (page 58).

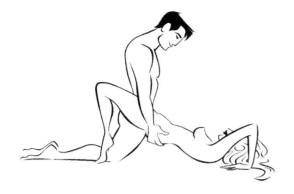

BRIDGING THE GAP

You're positioned on your back as in the Half Bridge (page 90) with your hips raised up toward your partner. Your legs are spread as in pelvic lifts.

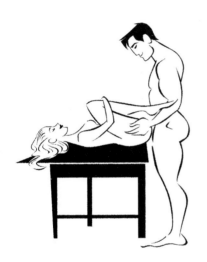

BUNDLED PACKAGE

In this position, known as the Wife of Indra in the *Kama Sutra,* your legs are tucked in like they are in the Wind-Relieving pose (page 120). Your partner takes hold of your hips and then penetrates. This is performed most easily with your partner standing at the edge of the bed and you scooted up to the edge of the mattress.

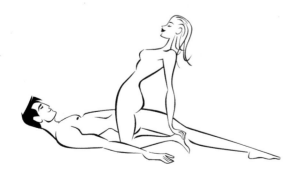

ORGASMIC CAMEL

Arch your back into a Camel position (page 62) holding your ankles while your partner lies underneath either performing oral sex or penetrating you.

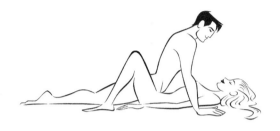

THE CONQUEST

Your partner is in the missionary pose with you underneath with your legs bent as in Bump Bump Bump (page 86). Raise your hips and perform some bumps to stimulate your man quickly.

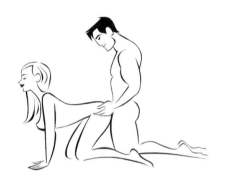

DOGGIE STYLE

You're in On All Fours (page 50) on your hands and knees while your partner enters you from behind.

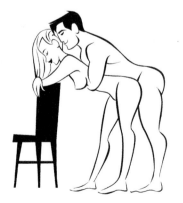

DOUBLE TRIANGLE

Stand in Reverse Triangle (page 154) with your hands on a wall or the back of a piece of furniture. Have your partner stand directly behind you, mimicking your posture, and then penetrating you.

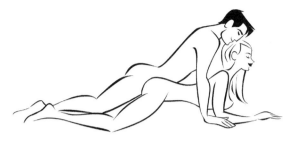

EROTIC FROGGIE

Start in On All Fours (page 50), then slide your knees outward into the Froggie (page 56). Your partner enters you from behind.

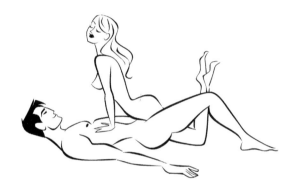

MERMAID

You're on top of your partner in Mermaid (page 64), he lies underneath with knees bent in Pelvic Squeezes (page 84), and both move hips to meet in the middle.

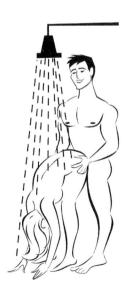

OOPS, I DROPPED THE SOAP!

Bend over fully with your hands placed firmly on the floor. Your partner stands behind and enters you. You can even try this out in the shower, but just make sure that your partner is holding you very carefully so that you don't slip and slide around.

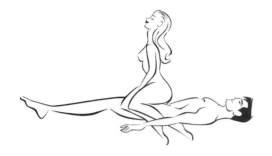

REARVIEW

Your partner lies on his back relaxing in At Peace (page 128). Sit on his lap while facing his feet.

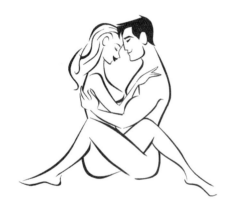

ROCK STEADY

You and your partner sit facing one another. Wrap your legs around each other's backs, as in a Butterfly pose (page 108), and steadily rock forward and back.

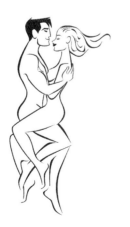

SATISFYING SIDE

Lie on your side, facing each other, with your legs entwined as in the Sexy Spinal Twist (page 110).

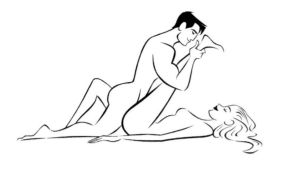

SPLITTING BAMBOO

Lie on your back with your partner on top. Raise one leg over the top of your lover's shoulders, as in Of Great Benefit (page 122) posture.

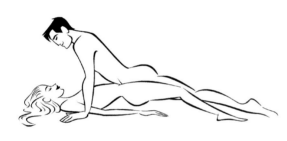

SURF'S UP

The Plank pose (page 44) looks like a surfboard when done properly. For this position, your partner is on top in Plank pose, with his upper body stiff and arms straight. Lie underneath with your legs slightly parted and move up and down to meet him.

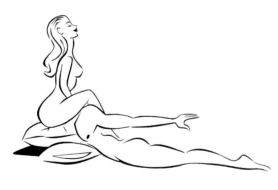

TALKING IN TONGUES

Lie down in Butterfly (page 108) with your back propped up on pillows while your partner performs oral sex. The giver is in a partial Locust (page 66) with back arched, in order for him to reach and pleasure you.

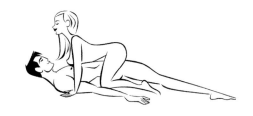

WILD CHILD

Your partner lies on his back while you mount on top on your knees in Sex Kitten position (page 52).

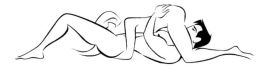

YIN YANG

Either you or your partner is on top while performing oral sex.

8

BEYOND BETTER SEX THROUGH YOGA

At this point we hope you've had a chance to experience the fabulous benefits of *Better Sex Through Yoga*. You've got a new toned, hot yoga body. You've put that new body to good use in the bedroom (and in the shower, and in the kitchen, and in the backseat of the car, you wild thing, you!). You're feeling great, you're looking hot, and you are having amazing sex. You're sexually satisfied, and so is your partner.

What else could be left to say? Mission accomplished, right? It can't get better than this . . . or could it? Could it turn out that there's even more to *Better Sex Through Yoga* than the best, wildest, hottest, most mind-blowing orgasmic sex you've ever had? Not possible, you say? But actually, it is.

Of course we're happy that you're experiencing more sexual pleasure. Unleashing your inner sex goddess (or for men, your inner Adonis) has been our goal, of course. But that's not our only goal. Better sex is an amazing, life-changing, thrilling, fabulous result of your faithful practice of the *Better Sex Through Yoga* routine, but there's a bigger picture too. Bigger even than the Big O.

Ultimately it all comes back to yoga—that was our starting point for the *Better Sex Through Yoga* program in the first place, and one of the main teachings of yoga is that true happiness comes from inside you. So yes, we want you to continue trying and experimenting with all of these great sexual positions and poses. But we also want to remind you not to lose sight of all the other wonderful and enlightening benefits of yoga.

Ultimately our wish for you is that your *Better Sex Through Yoga* practice goes beyond just feeling pleasure "down there." We want your *Better Sex Through Yoga* to help you with what's called "heart opening," so that your sexual energy doesn't just stay focused in your genital area but is fully integrated into your emotions and your life, allowing you to feel not just sexual satisfaction but satisfaction in all areas, experiences, and relationships.

Remember those chakras we talked about earlier? Your *Better Sex Through Yoga* practice has helped you to unclog and open the chakra related to your genital area, but yoga practice can do so much more—it can help you open your heart chakra. Great sex begins, after all, with an open heart. And an open heart is something you can carry with you not only in the bedroom, but everywhere throughout your life.

And speaking of your relationships, never forget to honor your partner. Don't just see your partner as a sexual object. Have the *Better Sex Through Yoga* experience be meaningful for both of you. Open your heart and bring your *Better Sex Through Yoga* practice—and your relationship—to a whole new level.

Have fun!

ACKNOWLEDGMENTS

The authors would jointly like to thank: Team Broadway; especially Ann Campbell, Laura Lee Mattingly, and Debra Manette; our agent, Lisa Queen, at the Queen Literary Agency; Lisa Hyman; Frank Montagna; and Eric Neuhaus, for his organizational mastery.

JACQUIE would like to thank: Garvey Rich, for his photographic genius and collaboration; all my teachers and dedicated students; Mom and Dad; and my loving husband, who provided continuous support and eagerness to enjoy all that yoga has to offer.

GARVEY would like to thank: The perfect complement and finisher of my thoughts and vision—Jacquie Greaux—may the Gyro always be with you; Mom and Dad, saved by the bell; Nidhi and John Huba, Lai Ling and Robert Clark; Alex di Suvero, Ken Scrudato, Carrie and Noe DeWitt; "A.J. here," A. J. Stetson; Dot and Frank; Amy Sohn; living proof that funny Germans exist, Andreas Troeger; Shiva Shala Patti and Adam for keeping me yoga sane or insane in NYC; Lang and Shane Hudepohl, life is a beach; Lynn and Michael Pelzman; Joel S. Berman; Warrior One Master Jason Hudepohl; Ron Burgundy; Aaron Star; David Lee for the never-ending supply of sexy leg warmers; Smarty and Meshugena; my loyal disciple and Tofu Honey Pie Rana Lee Araneta; El Diablo; Larisa and David Rich; Michael "it's the story that matters" Pagnotta; all present and future offspring have been omitted for the sake of decency. And last but not least, Barbara DeWitt—I miss you so.

JENNIFER would like to thank all of her friends, family, and mentors for their inspiration and support in writing this book. She could not have written this without the intelligent, artistic, and talented people she is so lucky to surround herself with everyday. She would especially like to thank Casey Moulton for his creative vision and guidance, Danielle Gelfand for her perpetual wit, Stephanie Edmonds for the unforgettable strolls of banter through the East Village, and Allie Abodeely for her infectious laughter—and all of you for your friendship and support. Thank you to my family—my heroes: Mom, for your creative genes and artistic vision; Dad, for your bold stance and quick-witted sense of humor; Tracie, for your values, and being someone I am proud to call my sister. Finally—thank you to everyone who has taught me the most valuable lesson of all—"everything you do, do with integrity."

Photographer: Garvey Rich, www.garveyrich.com

Equipment: RobertClarkPhoto.com

Lighting: Alex di Suvero

Clothing provided by: KD Dance, Stella McCartney, Adidas, and Nicko Noelle

Wardrobe: Keith Washington

Living Male Work of Art: A. J. Stetson @ AJStetson.com

Post-Production Consultant Master: JohnHuba.com

Digital: Canon 1Ds Mark II

Shot at: Berman's Improv Studio in NYC

JACQUIE NOELLE GREAUX Star instructor of the underground *Better Sex Through Yoga* DVD series, Jacquie Noelle Greaux is a San Francisco-based yoga instructor and massage therapist with over fifteen years of professional holistic healing experience. Yoga came to Jacquie at the early age of eighteen when she got hooked on its vast and powerful benefits. Since then, Jacquie has practiced with many of today's yoga masters, danced in the Houston Civic Ballet, and massaged American Olympic athletes. She is certified nationally and by the State of California as a teacher and practitioner of Oriental Body Therapy. Jacquie is also known for the pound-shedding, fantastic-tasting, and healthy meals that she cooks for private clientele in the Bay Area (LaRoutines.com). To contact Jacquie, please visit BetterSexThroughYoga.com.

JENNIFER LANGHELD Jennifer Langheld is a freelance television writer, producer, and director, who honed her talents at MTV producing on popular shows such as *The Tom Green Show, UnPlugged,* and *Live from the Ten Spot* concert series, as well as the *MTV Video Music Awards.* In recent years she has specialized in writing and developing TV pilots at various networks including SPIKE TV, VH1, Court TV, and Mark Burnett Productions.

Given her relentless travel schedule, Jennifer turns to fitness and yoga to maintain a healthy and balanced lifestyle. Jennifer currently resides in Los Angeles, where she is busy developing several projects including her lastest creation—a TV series about America's hot young entrepreneurs. Stay tuned.

GARVEY RICH Garvey Rich, professional photographer and director of the *Better Sex Through Yoga* video series, has been leading yoga-like stretching sessions even during his days warming up to play tackle football in grade school. He first studied yoga and dance at a children's acting workshop near his home in New York's Greenwich Village. He never fails to do some yoga every day and believes we are all gurus with something to learn from everyone.

Connecting with people via images, ideas, and word play is his passion. Past careers include being a flack for mega (and non-mega) stars in the music business and producing and casting high-end fashion photo shoots. Garvey resides in New York City's East Village. To contact Garvey, please visit BetterSexThroughYoga.com.